A Shallow Pool of Time

An HIV+ Woman Grapples
with the AIDS Epidemic

Fran Peavey

New Society Publishers

Philadelphia, PA   Santa Cruz, CA

Inquiries regarding requests to reprint all or part of *A Shallow Pool of Time* should be addressed to:

New Society Publishers
4527 Springfield Avenue
Philadelphia, PA 19143 USA

ISBN 0-86571-166-6 Hardcover
ISBN 0-86571-167-4 Paperback

Printed in the United States of America on partially recycled paper by BookCrafters, Fredericksburg, VA, USA.

Cover design by Rosa Lane.
Book design by Jana Janus and Mary Goodell.

To order directly from the publisher, add \$1.75 to the price for the first copy, \$.50 each additional copy. Send check or money order to:

New Society Publishers
PO Box 582
Santa Cruz, CA 95061 USA

New Society Publishers is a project of the New Society Educational Foundation, a nonprofit, tax-exempt, public foundation. Opinions expressed in this book do not necessarily represent positions of the New Society Educational Foundation.

Contents

Introduction

You will meet my friend Fran Peavey in these pages. Maybe you will also meet her in person some day at one of her performances or in connection with a social-change project. It is hard to tell what such a project would be, because Fran is the least predictable person I know. I gave up long ago trying to guess where that mind and heart of hers will take her. She refuses to be typecast, and, indeed, given her range of roles and activities it is pretty hard to do that.

To many, in devoted, uproarious audiences across the country and overseas, she is a stand-up comedian. She is the Atomic Comic who helps us confront the fearful dangers of our time and, by laughing at ourselves, break through apathy and despair. For laughter, like tears, recalls us to our common humanity and our power to change.

To men, women, and children in Benares, India, she is the faithful American friend who has helped them rally to clean up the disease-bearing pollution of Mother Ganga, the sacred river Ganges. Every year she comes back to listen, cajole, inspire, and serve as mirror to what they have accomplished in the intervening months.

To homeless alcoholics in the Tenderloin district of her city, she is the loud-voiced, straight-talking ally who worked with them to create the "Wino Park." Joking, scolding, encouraging, goading, she helped them carve out and beautify a piece of turf that was both a challenge and monument to their intrinsic dignity.

To readers around the world, she is the cheerful, ingenious companion they gained through her book *Heart Politics*. Its pages pull together many of her multifarious activities and reveal their common strands—compassion and humor and a dogged belief in humanity.

It was while writing *Heart Politics* in 1984 that Fran Peavey began taking notes on an unprecedented epidemic, notes that became her diary on AIDS. Charlie Varon, who at the time was a co-worker on the book as well as on the nuclear comedy show, noticed her making occasional entries in that file. "This is really happening, this AIDS epidemic," she explained. "It will be interesting to keep track of it over time, and interesting to people in the future—just as it would be for us to have a journal of an ordinary person who lived during the Plague."

"My first reaction," Charlie says, "was 'there goes crazy Fran again.' It seemed completely nuts and completely consistent." While it struck him as "another of her crazy ideas," he also knew of her long-standing fascination with the dynamics of a society under stress and with the kind of social breakdown and hysteria that happened with the Plague.

The diary, as it progressed over the next four years, recorded what she saw happening in the world around her and what she found erupting in her own most intimate life.

Recently Fran showed this diary to some of her friends. While each of us wanted to respect her privacy, at some deep level we knew that this remarkable document should be shared with a wider public. We sensed that it could play a critical role in building understanding and solidarity in a time of panic. It could dispel the ignorance on which panic feeds, and replace fear and divisiveness with sanity and trust. So Fran, out of the hugeness of her heart, decided to publish.

As I said, she can't be typecast. She can't be pigeonholed. She can no more be reduced to one role or activity than can you. Therefore, let yourself meet in these pages, not just a spokesperson for the HIV-afflicted, but a many-faceted friend, who shares with you her honesty and her courage.

Joanna Macy

Preface

I decided to begin a journal on the AIDS epidemic after a routine visit to a clinic sometime in 1984. In the small talk that occurs between doctor and patient, the topic shifted to AIDS, and my doctor expressed utter terror about the magnitude of the epidemic. I had never heard a doctor talk like this, and I remember thinking, "If the doctors are afraid, what is really going on?" It frightened me—not for myself, but for my society.

As a consultant on social change and a political comedian, I have tried to understand the social effects of the impending terrors of our time: ecological degradation, the possibility of economic collapse, and nuclear holocaust. Listening to this doctor, I sensed that the AIDS epidemic carried the same potential as these for invoking social hysteria. I have long been interested in this phenomenon—in what happens when an entire society gets scared. I know that, during the Black Plague, the social order dissolved into ugliness and hysteria. And yet I have also heard stories of nobility and generosity in those times.

I began to wish I could read the diary of a woman who lived in the time of the Plague. I've often thought, "If we are living in a time of rapid, unpredictable change and seeming social breakdown, what can we learn from those who have been through this in the past?" What clues could ordinary people—not kings, scientists, or states-men—give us about what to watch for as the epidemic begins to affect our community, family, relationships? What could we learn about keeping our focus in the midst of grief and confusion? About grieving and working and loving all in the same moment? The disruption of daily life must be analogous to that of war, I suspected. But then again, it must be different because an epidemic spreads so quietly.

So I decided to start a journal, a personal chronicle of the AIDS epidemic, as it affected my society, as it affected me. I thought it would be interesting to do, and I try to do only interesting things. It was not a very serious effort, so unfortunately, many specifics like dates and precise details were left out. But I fantasized that I would place the journal in an archive, where it would be available to people in the future who were facing epidemics of their own.

For the first few years my entries were sporadic. I would read something in the newspaper, or talk about AIDS with a friend, and record my impressions. Then in the spring of 1988, when I found out I was "with virus," the journal became a confidant. It helped me to pass through the morass of shocking information and sort things out. The writing was confused and often too detailed to interest anyone but me. But the process helped me reflect on events that were sweeping me along.

When dark days came to me that fall, I tired of trying to find words to explain to friends what was going on with me. I hit upon the idea of printing out the computer file containing these notes, just to share with a few long-time friends. I never dreamed of sharing it more widely.

The first two or three people who read it strongly encouraged me to publish. Although I was reluctant, I was in such a state of confusion that I welcomed any clear direction. I was upset about the political scene regarding AIDS (as evidenced by several bigoted propositions on the California ballot and in the U.S. Congress). If there was any way to move things along by helping people to see the world through HIV+ eyes, I would do it.

The decision to publish these highly personal reflections has not been an easy one to make. It is tough to be so vulnerable in print, and in many ways I am a different person now than when I began the journal.

Reading over the early entries, I am embarrassed by my prejudice, especially toward gay men, and by my uncaring attitude toward friends of mine who suffered early in the history of the disease. My alienation from intravenous drug users is evident. In reflecting on those entries that now seem arrogant and judgmental, I realize that there existed in my mind a "hierarchy" of AIDS victims. In other words, some people were more genuinely victims of the disease, while others "deserved" to be afflicted. I felt much less sympathetic toward gay men who had not used safe sex and toward IV drug users. I think this is a fairly common attitude. It is both tragic and terribly wrong that people already marginalized and oppressed by society are not seen as victims. No one should suffer this disease— or the shame and self-blame that occur as a result of social ostracism. No one deliberately brought this suffering on him- or herself.

Reacquainting myself with the journal to get it ready for publication, I was shocked at how confusing the entries were, beginning in mid-May of 1988. Considerable work was needed to make them readable. My friend Max Heirich came in from out of town and

helped organize a group to support me in this effort. In my friendship network, people were found to raise funds for the original
printing (Catherine and Jim Porter), to edit (Jan Thomas and Melissa
Everett) and design the book (Mary Goodell and Jana Janus), to
design the book cover (Rosa Lane), and to help me think strategically
(Joanna Macy, Michael Phillips, and Bob Fuller). Charlie Varon,
Terry Kelly, John White, and Carol Hale were also very helpful at
key moments.

Just when I thought the book was done, Jan Thomas began to
lobby for some more theoretical chapters, and especially for the one
on social hysteria. She knows me to be mind as well as heart. But this
assignment proved harder than it should be for me, a consultant on
social change. I kept saying, "I don't know what I know." So Jan and
Joanna spent a lovely fall Saturday afternoon dragging it out of me.

I debated until the last minute about whether to put my name on
this book. I consulted with other authors who had written controversial books. When I asked Nancy Manahan (*Lesbian Nuns: Breaking
Silence*), "Why did you publish under your own name?" she an-
swered, "Ego, pure ego." I guess this is my answer, too. This is the
life I have lived. Nancy also reminded me of the importance of
breaking silence. For in the AIDS crisis, it is silence which allows
bigotry to thrive, funding for research to be denied, and lives to be
lost.

I have relished much of the final writing, and am grateful to my
friends for suggesting that I do it. I have especially enjoyed the
solitary aspects of the project, and have been able to sneak words
into print that I know Charlie and Myra (who helped me write *Heart
Politics*) would never have let through. I end this writing project very
grateful to both of them for teaching me to write and encouraging me
to do it.

Many others have also helped this book find its way into your
hands and to them I am grateful. Ginger Ashworth, Patricia Averill,
Beverly Axelrod, Rosemary Ball, Patricia Bauer, Timothy Berke,
Sherpherd Bliss, Carl Buelow, Catherine Campbell, Mark Cantzler,
Alex Captanian, Jill Croucher and Sylvia Perez, Kathy Dennison,
Carol Goodman, Barbara Green, Tova Green, Lynn Griffis, Karen
Hagberg and Gail Seneca, Jeff Hasner, Barbara Hazard, Virginia
Hedelund, David Hoffman and Sharon Nelson, Gene Hoffman, Ann
Peavey Hoffer, Polly Howells, John and Susan Peavey Houth, David
Jenkins, Cynthia Jurs, Jon Katz, Thomas Kincaid, Maria Kerschen,
Brooke Kuhlman, Jenny Ladd, Monica Levin, Peggy Macy, Nancy
Manahan, C.J. Maupin, Stephanie Merrin, Mary Merwin, Dick Mayo-
Smith, Evelyn Messinger and Kim Spencer, Todd Nachowitz, Ferne
Orcutt, Arthur O'Donnell, Margaret Pavel, Art Peavey, Christine
Pelosi, Catherine Porter, Jim and Dee Porter, Dean Robb, Mimi

Rosenn, Betsy Rose and David Stark, Mary Sawyer, Blanche Streeter, Geraldine Simkins, Barden Stevenot, Carlene Waldrum, David Ward, Mark Weinrod, Yuri Wellington, Emma Williams, and the men and women in my HIV+ support groups who are nameless here but not to each other.

And of course special thanks to the folks at New Society Publishers who work so hard to make progressive and thoughtful books available to all of us. Especially I would thank Ellen Sawislak, David Albert, Barbara Hirshkowitz, and T. L. Hill.

Countless others whose names I do not know cut the trees, manufactured this paper and ink, designed the print typeface, printed this book, and delivered it into your hands. To them I am grateful. And to the trees whose life now joins mine, I bow.

A IDS has been a real "learning opportunity," as we say in the '80s, and for that I am grateful. It has brought me much closer to gay men and lesbians, and to people who have been IV drug users. It has helped me explore new dimensions of the peril we all face. I have learned a great deal about what an epidemic looks like from the inside: the urgency, the deep despair and rage, the persistent denial in myself and in society, as well as the decency and courage of many people in the face of catastrophe.

If you are one of the people who only know AIDS and HIV through the headlines of the newspaper, I hope you will meet people in this book who will challenge your assumptions about "what kind of people" get AIDS. This book is written for you. The face of destiny which gives some of us AIDS is the same one that brings us other kinds of pain: suffering due to hunger or war, the loss of love, the death of loved ones, helplessness experienced in the face of natural disasters. Some people suffer in illness and pain, others in health. But many aspects of suffering unite us. Sometimes gifts spin off from suffering, such as learning to be brave when we are afraid, finding strength in the midst of our weakness, being wise although we flounder in confusion, and surrendering when we can no longer hold on to that which we most covet. We learn vulnerability, courage and wisdom from our struggles. I hope, too, that this book will help you understand more clearly the responsibility we all share in stopping this epidemic and protecting the civil rights of those suffering in it.

If you are reading this book because you care about someone who is HIV+, I hope you will find in these pages tools to help you understand yourself and your friend. We are going to make many mistakes as we learn to live with this new disease. I hope you find light from my mistakes and those of my friends. In these pages I also hope you will find compassion for yourself in facing and learning from your mistakes. For you, too, are having to let go of dear ones and parts of their lives. I think I speak for all HIV+ people in saying how grateful we are for your caring and your willingness to stand with us. Sometimes we may find the differences in our options and situations worthy of righteous anger. But under that anger and frustration is a deep underground river of gratitude for whatever steadiness and calm you can bring to the raging torrents of our lives. Through the pages of this book I hope you will find the will not only to care for us, but to also to fight politically for our lives. And as we work together, it is clear that "we all have AIDS" in the society.

If you are one of more than a million people in the USA (or the five to ten million people worldwide) who are HIV+, I hope you will be reminded by this book that you are not alone. When you sweat at night in your bed and shake uncontrollably, know you are not alone. When you must die the little deaths, when you must let go of what you can no longer hold, you are not alone. This book was written for you—and for me, so that I can know that I am not alone.

When we look at each other's faces—the healthy, the afflicted—we see the face of destiny and humanity in all its toughness and fragility. We can teach each other so much in this time. In this difficult age, no one comes to the table of this moment empty handed.

Journal Entries
1984–1987

1984—AIDS is mostly a disease of gay men, although I hear that others can get it too. AIDS attacks the immune system. Sometimes AIDS, also known as GRID, is referred to as "gay cancer." Little splotches appear—that is the way it is diagnosed. It seems that this disease is spread by sex and that one gets it from bathhouses where gay men do things that I cannot imagine. It seems sad that something as intimate and fun as sex is getting such a bad reputation these days from sexually transmitted diseases (they're calling them STDs), such as herpes and now AIDS. Herpes is so important that it has been on the cover of *Time* magazine, but AIDS has not yet been a cover story in major media.

From what I hear and piece together from snatched fragments of conversations, gay men who frequent the bathhouses have sex many times in one night and with people they don't even know. I really don't know what it is like in these bathhouses. I hear about "glory holes," which are holes in toilet walls where I imagine someone puts his penis and someone on the other side plays with it and puts it wherever he wants to put it. I must confess that it kind of boggles my mind how someone could do that. I can only conclude that I must not understand this kind of gay male sexual pleasuring very well. I read in the gay press, however, that the behavior in the bathhouses is very controversial, and that many gay men are embarrassed and critical of anonymous sex without relationship.

Anyway, there is a lot of conversation about AIDS and whether or not they should close the bathhouses. It is a constitutional issue as well as a public health one. I read in the paper that the bathhouse owners are dispensing condoms and have posted guidelines every-where about safe sex. The other day one of the gay papers mentioned that someone showed up in the bathhouse with red AIDS blotches all over his body, and everyone freaked out.

But the gay papers are screaming about the attacks on the bath-houses and their freedom to express their sexuality any way they want. It is pretty confusing. Silverman, the city official in charge of public health, is trying hard to get the gay community's cooperation with his plan to close the bathhouses, but there is tremendous resistance within the gay business community and the gay press. Silverman says that unless the community agrees to closing them, dangerous sexual activity will continue to take place in the bath-houses, or it will simply go underground. As a result, the disease will spread. It is a pretty confusing issue to figure out.

Spring 1984—My roommate Nancy, who works as a nurse, came home very late today. She had pricked her finger with a needle and had to stay and fill out a number of forms. Anyone on the hospital staff who is exposed to blood pricks must do this now because of AIDS.

Occasionally I read in the paper about nurses who refuse to care for AIDS patients. Nancy is furious at these nurses. She says, "We have a very active nursing education program teaching us how to change our practices to handle this epidemic, and those who refuse to treat patients are just ignorant." She feels ashamed of her profession. Some nurses are even quitting because they are afraid of catching AIDS.

December 1984—My friend Dennis, a gay medical student in New York, says that AIDS is going to be the biggest epidemic of our time. He is confident that he won't get it. But the story he painted of the disease was of people withering away, losing their minds, and dying young and vital. It is upsetting him a lot. He thinks that the govern-ment may have invented this disease as a form of biological warfare, and is now using it to get rid of gay men because they threaten the male power structure.

On a recent visit, as we sat talking under cherry blossoms, he told me about an experience he had last year. A casual acquaintance—actually his upstairs neighbor—came down in the middle of the night to show Dennis some marks which had appeared on his body. The neighbor wanted to know if he had AIDS. Dennis said he probably did. He told me this in a taut professional tone that barely masked his fear. Almost all he's talked about on his last visits has been AIDS and his concern about what is happening to the gay community.

I listened to him ramble and wondered if he's right, if AIDS is really such a big problem. How can I tell?

January 1985—Got a postcard from Dennis. It arrived on a very busy day, and I read it quickly. He has pneumonia. It seems odd that he would make it a point to write me about it.

Several months later—I visited Dennis last week in New York. In the middle of our conversation, I asked him about his pneumonia. Slowly it came out that he has AIDS. I asked him, "Was that what you were trying to tell me in that postcard?" He said, "Yes." I was so ashamed that I had not responded to the card—I had been either too busy or too ignorant to feel the impact of the information. Or perhaps it was because he had used the scientific term, "pneumocystic pneumonia," which is not in my regular vocabulary. I told him how horrible I felt that I hadn't understood and responded to his card. "How did you feel when I didn't call or write?" I asked. "It doesn't really matter now," he replied wearily, and I knew I had hurt him. We looked at each other for a moment, then let go and moved on.

I asked him if it meant he was going to die. He said very definitely, "No." I said "Okay," and stopped worrying. But now as I write this, there is a corner of concern in my mind. How can he be sure?

There is a lot that I just don't know about AIDS.

When I told Dennis about my social change work, he said almost pleadingly, "Why don't you figure out what to do about AIDS? We need some big changes if we are to keep so many people from dying." I thought about it for a minute, but didn't really see what I could do. How frustrating it is not to be able to help my friend.

Summer 1985—There is a diet product on the market called AYDS. They used to advertise it all the time, but now people laugh when they hear on the radio about how AYDS helps people lose weight. AIDS is also known as the wasting disease, because the people who have it become so gaunt and thin.

Fall 1985—Every now and then I read about a doctor refusing to take patients with AIDS, saying they have to consider their families. Nurses occasionally quit hospitals if they are forced to treat AIDS patients. It's really coming down now. There is a shortage of rubber gloves. Medical and dental health care workers are supposed to be wearing them; and police wear them when they arrest people in demonstrations. Ambulance attendants wear them all the time. Sometimes I feel crazy kissing gay men at church. The virus has been found in saliva and tears, I hear. The medical insurance establishment is saying that they may go broke because of AIDS patients, and they are trying to figure out how to refuse insurance to them. If you are an unmarried male, they just don't want your money now, thank you.

Fall Tour, 1985—Riding in a taxi in New York on my way to see Dennis with Carol, my "social change apprentice," we chatted about AIDS. Carol's father is gay and she has some anti-gay sentiments although she herself is a lesbian. We talked about these issues for quite a while before getting to Dennis's place. The cab driver, a black man, joined our discussion. He told us he was from Haiti. "We are always getting the blame for this AIDS mess," he complained. "My daughter came home from school the other day saying the kids were bugging her, saying that our people were AIDS people. She was in tears." He said rarely does a week go by now but what someone in his cab or elsewhere mentions his Haitian background and AIDS in the same breath. "I'm tired of being blamed for this disease. I don't have it and it's not my fault. It's racism...that's what it is. It's just another way for them to blame everything on us."

We met Dennis and his lover Mark at their modest but beautiful apartment. Dennis looks strong and vibrant. Before we went out to dinner, I had to use the toilet, but I was worried about whether the seat might be infected. I apologized to Dennis; still, I had to ask. He laughed and said the virus can't be transmitted by toilet seats, and besides he uses the bathroom near their bedroom. I should not worry.

There was no mention of AIDS during dinner. At one point, Carol's and Dennis's water glasses became confused. It was an awkward moment because of fear of drinking out of the "wrong" glass, and I was frozen with fear. Dennis ordered two fresh glasses. I thought he handled it elegantly. Turns out that he was as concerned about getting bugs that Carol might have had and introducing them into his weak system as she was about getting AIDS from his glass. He laughed later when we talked about this, saying she was safer in that situation than he was.

After dinner we walked several blocks to the bus and Mark strolled with Carol, giving Dennis and me a chance to talk alone. Dennis told me how much Mark's love meant to him these days. He told me that Mark had requested a change in his residency schedule so he could sleep nights with Dennis when he was ill in the hospital. Although Mark didn't have to take on the stigma of Dennis's AIDS at his work place, he did so to be with Dennis. I admired Mark and was grateful for the love he was giving my dear friend.

Dennis said he was determined to "beat this thing." I said that to my way of thinking, the victory was in how you handled whatever came along, not just winning the length-of-life battle. Victory could well be getting through this time in a friendly and gracious way, letting people love you, staying real through whatever came. In other words, refusing to give into pretense or bullshit. To me, that is the victory in every day—including your last one. Dennis held tightly to the belief that he was going to "beat this thing."

Dennis talked about how great Mark was to stay by him and how much he had learned about love from Mark. He also complained about the hospital's having fired him. He is suing for compensation.

We gave each other a long and intense hug when we said goodbye. I don't know if I will ever see him again.

Looking back, I don't think I was completely supportive of Dennis in feeling that his firing was unjust. I am at least ambivalent about having a doctor with AIDS. I don't know if there is any threat, but I think I might be concerned about it. I need to find out more about how AIDS is really spread. But who do I believe? The government that has lied to me about all the major issues of my time, from Vietnam to Three Mile Island to toxic pesticides? Still, I should find out more.

Fall 1985—I had lunch with my friend Chris at a Korean restaurant. He is gay. For two hours he talked about AIDS. In the past month, twelve of his friends have died. What would that mean in my life if twelve of my friends vanished? I was horrified. He thinks it is a plot or some man-made virus that escaped from a laboratory somewhere. All he could talk about during lunch was AIDS. He is completely preoccupied. It must be like the holocaust for him, losing so many people. I am starting to wonder what I should do.

Spring 1986—I had a middle-aged white man in my cab the other day. He asked me to show him some of the sights on the way to the airport, so we were together for longer than usual. He asked me about the "queers" in the city. He had noticed them and had been very uncomfortable. He said a few other things ending with, "Don't you wonder about this disease being God's punishment to them for being so promiscuous and sinful?" I said, "No." Then I took a minute or two to think about how to respond to this guy. He was from Oklahoma and probably didn't know any better. I told him how hard the disease was on this community and how deep their suffering was. I told him about Chris losing so many friends in one month. I also said that gay people are a minority in their own families, and that it is terribly hard for them to be hidden, to live shadow lives.

Now it was his turn to be quiet. As we turned on the airport off-ramp from the freeway, he said, "I have a boy. He might grow up to be gay. How can I tell? I wouldn't want him to think I didn't approve of him if he was. I would want him to know I loved him no matter what he was."

July 1986—On my way to South Africa, I called Dennis from the airport in New York. He sounded terrible. Could hardly speak.

Stumbled with long pauses as he tried to form each word and thought. Sounded aphasic. Had he had a stroke or what? I wondered if I should call Mark. He said no. He said he was having trouble talking. He has a long "pozie" on his nose which he talked about a long time. I'm not sure what a pozie is, but I think it is some kind of mark associated with AIDS.

August 1986—A few weeks ago I decided to take the AIDS test. I'd been wondering for some time about whether or not to do it. When I had those blood transfusions early in the decade, I surely drew from the San Francisco blood pool. My friend Rita was tested and encouraged me to do likewise. (She was scared to death, as she'd been dating San Francisco men for ten years.)

I've heard of a nun who died of AIDS from a transfusion. Did I want to know if I was carrying the virus? That was the big question. What would I do if the test came back positive? What impact would that have on my life?

The question of whether or not to take the test is very controversial. Some people say that since there is no cure or treatment, there is no reason to be tested; a positive result will only bum you out. Others say you should know so you won't be tempted to engage in unsafe sex.

Anyway, the *Bay Guardian* runs ads for AIDS testing, so I called the number and made an appointment. They said they'd had a cancellation for this Thursday; otherwise there was a waiting list of three weeks. So, in a burst of bravado, I agreed to the Thursday appointment. They asked me for a letter/number code by which I would be known throughout this process to ensure my anonymity. I made up something which I hoped I wouldn't forget and wrote the date and time in my appointment book.

Two weeks later—Well, Thursday came and went with no AIDS test for me. It was an unconscious decision—I rarely miss appointments that I've written in my book. I don't know if I'm sorry or not. Clearly, I don't seem to be in a rush to make another appointment. Besides, I don't think the result would be positive anyway; I'm very healthy and have a body which doesn't even catch colds. My immune system doesn't seem to be under attack.

Summer 1986—Reading the *Bay Area Reporter*, a San Francisco gay weekly, I was struck by all the obituaries in the current issue. Eight in one week! Although I don't read this paper regularly, I don't remember seeing obituaries in it before, and now there are so many. They were beautifully written. Usually they include a little about the man's life—where he used to hang out, what he liked to do, who would be missing him, and whether his lover was with him when he died. Most of them say that he died of "AIDS or AIDS-related conditions." It's becoming a little more real to me. This many people lost in one week in one community. I have read about people who have lost most of their friends. This is really an epidemic.

Summer 1986—Eating dinner with my brother in a fancy restaurant last month, I watched as he leaned over the table and said confidentially, "Don't you think that AIDS is a fitting punishment for what the gays have been doing all these years?" I said as calmly as possible, "No, I don't think so. First of all, the torture and suffering of AIDS could only fit a crime more awful than I can imagine. Secondly, I don't really think what they have been doing is such a crime."

It was a major disagreement. He still lives in Idaho where he thinks there are no homosexual people. He is sure of this. I understand where his prejudice comes from, but that doesn't make it any less painful when I think of my good friends who are gay.

He knows of a large international industrial company that burned all the furniture in their office when they found out that one of their employees had AIDS. And of course they fired him. My brother doesn't even find that bizarre.

It's maddening to know and love someone in my own family who is so uneducated about gay people, many of whom he would like if he knew them. For instance, I know he would like Chris and Dennis. My brother is not mean-spirited, but it is sometimes hard to remember that his attitude results from lack of social exposure more than anything.

Yet there is something else. The alienation of straight people from gay is often expressed in terms of hatred. People cling to this hatred, but why? What is it we learned to make us so fearful of the unknown? There is deep, alienating pain in those who hold attitudes like my brother's, and I don't know how to help people to unlearn their prejudice.

My first response upon coming to San Francisco from Idaho in the early 1960s and learning that people were sometimes attracted to people of their own gender was, "Well, it's logical. If you flip two coins, sometimes they'll be heads and heads, sometimes tails and tails, and sometimes heads and tails. One shouldn't expect that men will love only women, or women only men." I saw homosexuality as a statistical imperative. Now in my own life, I have found my way to being an "equal opportunity lover."

In this discussion with my brother, our real differences were visible. Although it was a quiet fight (unlike some of our political fights which tend to be screaming, teasing, and fun-loving), this one hurt ever so softly, and left many bruises.

Fall 1986—Today I heard a report on television about foster parents who are willing to care for babies born with AIDS. The mothers of these babies are mostly intravenous (IV) drug users who can't cope with a newborn infant as they fight for their own lives. Someone has to care for these babies until they die. The report also mentioned that they might not all die. What heroes of this time are the people who pour their love on these little AIDS babies!

I'll bet the life expectancy in this country is going to drop soon due to this epidemic.

Fall 1986—I've been thinking about building a community hot tub in my backyard. I want a hot tub for myself and it seems like a waste for only one person to use it. So I made a list of who on the block might be interested. Then I came upon the question of the guys across the street. I like them and they would probably want to be included. What if they have AIDS? Can AIDS be spread in hot tubs? How can I tell? Does anyone know the answer? Oh dear, another point where I have to make a decision which could be oppressive to two fine people, based on simple lack of information. Well, maybe I'll do nothing for a while and see if I come across any new information.

Winter 1986—Bob, the man with whom I work on a number of social change projects, and I traveled to the Afghan refugee camps in Pakistan last month. We went to research the situation for some speaking engagements. I was particularly interested in the conditions of women refugees. With this trip, I had to come to grips with the Soviet invasion of Afghanistan. Actually, at this point both the Soviet invasion of Afghanistan and the AIDS invasion in San Francisco have been going on about the same length of time. I haven't been very outspoken against the Soviet invasion, and in talking with the Mujaideen (Afghan liberation fighters), I was stunned to learn of the level of killing and nastiness that the Soviets were committing in their country. The Mujaideen impressed me with their determination, loyalty, and independent spirit.

While going through a Red Cross hospital there I was confronted with so many people, not only men but women and children, who had lost arms and legs. People more seriously wounded die in the field because the nearest hospital is two to four days from the battlefield. They asked if I could give blood, as I was obviously well nourished and strong. Of course I agreed and was taken down the hall where I was introduced to the blood-drawing team. They were a friendly group who were amazed to see an American woman out alone in this place. They asked me about past illnesses, very much as they do in the Red Cross blood banks here.

Out of curiosity, I inquired if they had the capacity to test blood for AIDS and how that was affecting their blood pool. They looked stunned and shortly left the room for a consultation with someone. The head nurse returned with them and asked if I had reason to believe that I had AIDS. I said no, but I could see doubt on their faces. Nevertheless, I left my blood there and am proud that it is probably now either inside an Afghan or spilled on a battlefield.

My co-workers, members of the Mo Tzu organization for social change, have since been critical of me for being so cavalier about giving my blood. They know there is some risk that I could have gotten the virus in the transfusions I have received. I promised to get my AIDS test before donating blood again. In fact, we decided we all should take the test as a measure of security since we have all lived and dated in San Francisco for years. Also, taking the AIDS test confirms in a deep way that we live in the 1980s. We even laughed at our own denial in this matter.

I have had a number of transfusions in the last ten years, all from the San Francisco blood pool. That is really the only way I could have gotten the AIDS virus unless my one sexual experience with Dennis in 1973 gave it to me. But I don't think that the disease was invented then.

January 1987—I was working in New York last week and called Mark to ask if I could visit Dennis. He said that Dennis is not doing so well. He can't talk and has difficulty walking. He has expressive aphasia, as opposed to total aphasia. In other words, he can understand language and read, but he can't produce intelligent sound.

Mark invited me to dinner the next night. When I arrived, Dennis was sitting in an easy chair, reading *Time* magazine. He seemed glad to see me. I carried on a one-way conversation; he could communicate "yes" and "no." At one point he got up to go to the toilet. Mark helped him, as he could hardly walk. I watched, feeling useless and awkward, embarrassed that he should have to have me see him like this. I was filled with awe at how these two fine men make their life work.

Mark told me that Dennis had recently visited his parents and that since then his mother calls nearly every day. It seems that she and his father have made peace with the reality of Dennis's life and illness. Previously they had refused to allow Dennis to come home for his brother's graduation because of his AIDS. This had hurt Dennis very much.

At dinner Dennis got very angry at Mark for giving him only half of the chocolate cake rabbit I had brought for him. How frustrating to have people who can talk have complete power over your life.

Mark gave him the whole rabbit when he realized what Dennis wanted, but I felt he was paternalistic in the negotiation. I am sure it's hard to remember that Dennis is not a child, but a grown and intelligent man. I spoke with Mark later about this.

Dennis went into the bedroom to lie down while Mark and I did the dishes and talked. Macho to the end, Mark swore they were going to "beat this" somehow. When I went into the bedroom to say good-bye to Dennis, tears welled up in my eyes. I sat on the bed and talked to him about our history—how we had been students together; how I appreciated him helping me with the computer class and getting me the data-entry position when I lost a summer job; how kind he had been to me in school. I also appreciated his relationship with Mark and how he had learned to love another person in such a beautiful way.

And then I told him how important he was to me and to the world. He had always said he wanted to be important. I used to argue with him, saying if he wasn't important right now, he would probably never be important. "Being important is something one carries around inside," I would tell him. It was a thread running through our conversations over the years.

We had first met in a doctoral program at UCLA in the late 'sixties where we were both on fellowships. Dennis was from North Carolina, with a southern accent and manner. People in our doctoral program tended to pick on him. We were required to take a class in what was then called "sensitivity training." Each week the class would focus their long critiques on Dennis. I never called them on this, even though I noticed that we spent a lot of time talking about Dennis, and that this said as much about us as it said about him. I sat quietly, the only antiwar protester (complete with red arm band) among the group, many of whom were in the military. I was shy, and deathly afraid they would start in on me. So I kept quiet or joked and tried to ease things along.

Looking back, perhaps this was appropriate to that situation. Blaming him seems inappropriate. I know that Dennis participated in the dynamic. He hadn't yet acknowledged openly that he was a gay man, and he never brought his lover to our parties. In saying good-bye to Dennis, however, the only thing that mattered was that I had not stood by him in those classes. I apologized to him for that. I also remembered that he had not done well on the exams, passing only provisionally, while I received some of the highest marks ever given. I had secretly gloated, knowing I was smarter and better liked by our peers, while outwardly trying to make him feel good. Oh, what bullshit! I am ashamed now as I think back on it all.

Last week, in a very different world, both of us different people, I sat on his deathbed crying for him and for my loss of an old friend.

I said straightforwardly, "I may not see you again. I want you to know how much I love you and how great I think you are." But my tears got in the way. He looked pained and embarrassed by the tears. I rubbed his feet as I talked. Then we hugged and I noticed he was trembling.

Mark was standing outside Dennis's room listening. As I left, he said in a chipper tone that they might see me soon in San Francisco—"Not to say good-bye, just for a little trip." I wished him well and said that I admired him for the way he was taking all this. Then I walked into the cold hall and outside, where it was dark and snowing. I knew I was losing someone valuable to me. Dennis was gone. Or going. It seemed inescapable to me now.

Spring 1987—I have had close gay friends for years. Who in the Bay Area doesn't? Ever since Fred died, after our two-and-a-half years together, and then after Lew and I broke up even though we loved each other dearly, I've considered myself an "equal opportunity lover." I found myself loving a woman not because I wanted to be part of a social movement, or cared about being "politically correct," but just because of her. It was an intensely personal choice, not a political one. In San Francisco's politics, people tend to be categorized—you're either gay or straight. I feel that I am both, open to loving whomever I choose to love. It seemed so simple at the time, and it still does. I've managed to live openly with lesbian relationships and gay friends in a predominantly heterosexual world, and I've never closed the door to another relationship with a man.

I've been attending a gay church, Metropolitan Community Church, for about three years now. Before that, I had made the Society of Friends (Quakers) my spiritual home. But I wanted to sing and make noise with other people, so I began shopping around. I felt at home right away at MCC. There were people there who, like me, had created their own sexual identity and lifestyle, as well as straight people. I reveled in the racial mixture, the organist in leather pants, and the celebration of sexuality as a positive aspect of life. My heart sang when we talked about our God loving everyone.

Frequently in church there is mention of AIDS. During community prayer someone prays for a negative test result, or the pastor mentions AIDS patients who are in the hospital or at home. Possibly because so many people in the congregation are facing life and death issues, MCC is a deeply nourishing spiritual community. But there is more than that. Possibly because the suffering of the congregation is so intense, the spiritual search has a vibrancy which contradicts that suffering. So many people there have been rejected by their families as a result of their decision to live according to the preferences they evidently came into this world with. So many—some 60 to 75 percent at this point, they say—are HIV+. They are forced by that status to grapple with issues of death, pain, and diminishment of life force. It is obvious upon walking into a service that these people are jubilantly alive. They care deeply for each other and are a real community.

Last Sunday I went to church for the first time in five months—partly because I forgot and partly because I was working in India and on comedy tour. The church was celebrating an anniversary. Howard Wells, the man who started the San Francisco congregation, was to preach. So I went.

The service progressed normally until Howard began his talk. He was a short, stocky, balding man wearing a business suit, with a Texas accent. He talked for a while about the history of MCC in San Francisco. Then he told us that in spring of last year he had learned that he was HIV positive, and soon after he was fighting for his life in the hospital. I think it was pneumonia. The entire church grew still. It was the first time I had ever seen anyone stand up in a public meeting and acknowledge being HIV positive.

He said, "I've learned that I have AIDS, but AIDS doesn't have me. I am more than this disease, and I've learned not to use AIDS as an excuse for being lazy or irresponsible. I also believe God loves me as much as He ever did." He said he was closer to his parents and family than ever before. His 60-year-old parents mow his lawn now because they are afraid something will happen to him. He joked about what the neighbors must think about a younger man letting his parents mow his lawn.

He carefully distinguished being healed from being cured. He was not sure he could be cured of AIDS, but he would consider himself healed, he said, if he could allow people to love him and if he could forgive those who have hurt him. He said that HIV-positive people can have a better, richer, and finer life, or they can just continue death-oriented behaviors and live worse lives. He spoke about having experienced a "restored Shalom" since finding he was HIV positive.

When he stopped talking, people stood up spontaneously. I looked around and saw a lot of wet cheeks. Someone had spoken a truth that needed to be heard. Supposedly around sixty men in the church are now HIV positive.

April 1987—Peter Jennings, the news broadcaster, was in San Francisco for a spacebridge my co-workers at Internews and I were doing with the Soviets, so he broadcast his nightly news program from here. One night he closed by saying that he was broadcasting from San Francisco and had toured AIDS treatment facilities here. Some footage of very sick people was shown, as Jennings met and talked to them. He described how our community is rallying to care for AIDS victims, and how many services and volunteers there are to help them. He said, "San Francisco is a city which has always taught America tolerance for people who are different—racially, politically, and in lifestyle. Now it is a city that is teaching us how to die."

I'm proud to be a San Franciscan, and so proud of my city and how we are handling this tragedy.

Journal Entries
1987–1988

"They are falling all around me"
—*Bernice Johnson Reagan*

April 30, 1987—A card announcing Dennis's death came today. It didn't surprise me, but I feel very sad. I shall miss him. There will be a memorial service for him at Riverside Church in a week or two. I wish I could go, but I cannot. I will try to write something for the service.

For My Friend Dennis

I thought that epidemics were for other people in other times.
But now I have lost a dear friend
   in our own epidemic
   in our own time.
He was a good man
   consistently kind to me and to everyone I saw with him.

Snatched away by some vile bug
   which has come to our planet in this time.
I don't pretend to understand much
   about why this is happening to us in our time,
   or why it should happen to such a fine person as Dennis
   or to the thousands of other fine people
   who are fighting this same snarling dragon.

All I know is that it is the challenge of our time
to remain decent to each other
in the most difficult of circumstances,
to love those who are going into that dark night of our epidemic
   fighting this dragon called AIDS,
and to continue to love those who are staying with us for a while
   longer
carrying on with love the battles of those who have gone before.

I learned a lot from Dennis
  and will always remember him.
  His laughing and gentle chiding
  when I fell short of his mark for me.
When I couldn't understand something which was easy for him
  he would teach me, then move on.
For his dignity—in the face of prejudice and difficulty
  he would remain steady and kind.

Good-bye, dear friend.
You always wanted to be an important person.
And you made it.

Petals of tears drop as I finish this last farewell.

But then maybe it is not the last farewell.
  Maybe somewhere
    someday
      I'll meet Dennis under some other cherry tree
        besides the one by the zoo
  where we sat only a few springs ago.
  The blossoms will be falling on us
  and we will know there is beauty again in the universe.

Several Weeks Later—Mark called to tell me about the memorial service. Dennis's parents came. My poem was read only after heated discussion among the family. It was the only mention in the entire service of how Dennis died, and his parents would have preferred that AIDS not be mentioned. Mark finally concluded the discussion by saying that I was a good friend of Dennis and also a "famous writer," and that my poem had to be read intact. I am proud that my poem brought the reality of AIDS into Dennis's service. I think it would have pleased him. It seems that they had a good time at the party afterward, which Dennis would have appreciated.

June 1987—I read the other day about a really remarkable change that has happened to the face of this epidemic. A group called the STOP A.I.D.S. project marshalled 7,000 volunteers to do community education and organizing. Since 1984 they have been promoting the use of safe sex practices in the gay men's community. They held house meetings with small groups and pioneered peer-counseling projects to change the sexual behavior of gay men. I would have doubted that their goals could have been accomplished, so entrenched and defended were the positions and practices they were dealing with. But fortunately, these were people who were more optimistic than I—and it has been achieved! Several studies now indicate that new cases among the San Francisco gay community have dropped to a negligible rate. Gay men really have made major changes in their lives. More and more I read that they are learning to value long-term relationships. And they are using condoms and eliminating dangerous behaviors. The real heroes of this epidemic include this group of volunteers who sallied forth to tilt at windmills and save a people. Each of the men who agreed to preserve his life and that of his partner is part of this change. Step-by-step, man by man, the tide may have been turned for these people. I sure hope so.

As if this were not enough, the group did another thing that I find really amazing. They have just announced that since they have achieved their goal, they are going out of business!

I took my cousin on a tour of Polk Street and the Castro the other day. She had lived on Polk Street when it was a center for a certain kind of leather gay population about ten years ago. Many of the businesses she remembered had closed, and street life in both areas was a fraction of what it had been. Now on Castro, some stores stand empty for months before someone comes in to open a shop. A different mood reigns on the street. People still move about, it's still friendly, but it's quieter and poorer. Money is going into keeping friends afloat, supporting organizations doing research, and community organizing. It is no longer the street of gaiety and hustle.

August 1987—I was meeting on business with Chris. The talk turned, as it always does with him, to AIDS. I asked him if he was positive. Rather firmly, he told me, "You don't ask people that these days. It is very personal, and people don't want to say. You can assume that most gay men in San Francisco are positive. But don't ask." So now I see a code of manners emerging from this epidemic. It establishes what one can and cannot ask another person. I am amazed at how even manners are affected.

Late August 1987—This month I was hospitalized with severe bleeding from my vagina. I have had chronic endometritis (an infection of the lining of the uterus, often confused with endometriosis which is very different) for many years, ever since I had a Dalkon shield inserted. I have been hospitalized for this condition four times in the past fifteen years. I was passing large pint-sized pieces of liver-like blood clots every fifteen minutes or so. The last two days I had been using handtowels instead of Kotex because nothing could handle the flow. Blood seemed everywhere.

In the hospital, nearly everyone who handled me wore gloves, and we talked about it. One man was not wearing gloves. When I asked him about it, he said in a macho kind of way, "I don't wear those things. It's too much bother. And I haven't had any problem yet anyway." He frightened me with his attitude. Maybe he doesn't have any problem with AIDS yet, but if he develops one, it won't be easily fixed. He doesn't seem to understand that. Or maybe he's unconsciously suicidal.

I had a D&C to stop the bleeding. They said I was very weak from the loss of blood, but they were not transfusing anyone now unless it was a matter of life and death. Blood was in short supply, and more to the point, possibly tainted with the AIDS virus. I was directed by the doctor to go home and make my own blood. It would be safer just to stay in bed.

I still don't have enough blood to stand up for any length of time. I'm on iron pills and taking it easy for a month. So here I am—a blood factory because of AIDS.

(I also heard again in the hospital that there is a nationwide shortage of rubber latex gloves.)

Early Fall 1987—I had to wait for my prescription to be filled at the hospital pharmacy yesterday. There is a little room where you wait watching a large board with many numbers printed on it. The number of your prescription lights up when it is ready, and then you go into another room to pick it up.

As I sat there looking up at the number board, I overheard a conversation between a man, his male friend, and his mother. He had just learned that he has AIDS, and he was grappling with this news right there in the prescription room. He would talk for about four or five minutes about how depressed he was, then he would wonder what he was going to do with his goldfish. He would return to the reality of his situation, then back to the tank and each kind of fish. Maybe he should just get rid of them now because they are so difficult to move and he loves them so much. But who would give them the kind of care he has been giving them? After discussing this for awhile, they would return to the problem of AIDS. In a macabre way I found this whole scene funny and couldn't help laughing inside.

Fall Tour 1987—On tour in northern Michigan, we were hosted by an old friend, Jim. His new wife is a campus pastor at a small community college in Traverse City, a little tourist town. She had to go to a meeting of the district that supervises her work. On the agenda was a move on the part of some committee members to ask her to step down from her position for two reasons: (1) she was divorced before marrying my friend, Jim; and (2) she was ministering to AIDS patients. Since gay people were not living "moral lives," they should not be ministered to.

Dee is a member of the Disciples of Christ Church, and it is shocking to see a mainline church still acting this way. If there is sin, it must include rejecting people for acting and living according to the identity God gave them. As if somehow they thought that God didn't love gay people! If God didn't love gay people, why did She make so many of them—and in every corner of the world?

I asked Dee how many AIDS victims exist in this community. "Five or six so far," she replied. To have met the virus in a town so far from the urban centers was shocking. AIDS must be everywhere now if it is so visible even in Traverse City. And the struggle for treatment and acceptance is everywhere as well. There must be thousands of people like Dee who, in their own way, are working against tremendous social odds.

I asked her what she does for the people with AIDS. She said that she raises money for AZT, food, and clothing, but mostly she counsels and sits with them when they are facing death.

Dee returned that evening from the battle with the committee, tired but victorious. The move to sack her has been stalled for the time being.

Fall 1987—It is the strangest thing, but I am beginning to miss people. Not anyone I knew personally, for the most part, but people who were always part of the neighborhood landscape. The two men in shorts at church are gone now. I don't know where they are. Joe Robertson isn't around anymore. Some of the regulars on the street have just disappeared. The change is almost imperceptible—it's as if the ghosts of these people are hovering around, reminding me that they're gone. Are they all dead? I don't know and can't figure out who or how to ask. I tried calling Joe once but got an answering machine, and he didn't return my call. So he must still be alive. But I have a very distinct feeling that people are just dropping out of existence.

October 1987—As I walked through my office at Internews this afternoon, I noticed Maria was crying. Maria manages the office and has lots of spunk and good energy. I overheard her talking about a friend who is dying of AIDS. The man she works for asked if she wanted to take the day off, but Maria replied that this is a continuing pain. Today was no worse than any other day.

If this epidemic continues to grow as they say it might, it is going to affect the work force of this country dramatically. A mourning work force is not a very productive one. AIDS could have serious implications for industrial policy. For instance, just as many companies have discovered that providing a nursery for workers' children ensures a more reliable work force, the workplace of the future may also have to provide a care center for adults who are so ill that their partners or parents need to be near them during the day.

An epidemic hurts everything—including the workplace. Sooner or later those who are concerned about our nation's productivity must begin to pressure the government to put more effort into research for a cure or, at least, effective means of prevention.

Winter 1987—I heard a wonderful story about a group in the Bay Area that takes care of the animals of AIDS patients. When the person with AIDS (now known as PWA in the new language that has emerged from this epidemic) is no longer strong enough to care for a pet, this group finds someone to do it. The volunteers feed pets, walk dogs, clean bird cages, or do whatever else needs to be done. This allows the pet to stay with the owner until the very last, and the volunteer promises to find a good home for it after the owner dies.

Little things like this bring home the many ways that this epidemic has affected our everyday lives, and how our community has risen to respond to this challenge. It reassures me that human beings will take care of everything in other kinds of disasters as well, if given the time.

Christmas 1987—Last Sunday I went to see the quilt put together by the Names Project. I pulled up to Moscone Center and saw a line stretching out the door, down to the corner, around the block (which includes essentially two city blocks!), around the second corner, and halfway down the third block. This was the Sunday before Christmas when one expects most people to be busy with shopping and parties. It was a quiet group, with no hawkers or street vendors around.

People walked to the back of the line with looks of amazement at the number of people ahead of them. The crowd was a cross-section from practically the whole Bay Area—Black, white, Asian, Latin, gay, straight, young, old, middle-aged. The only group missing seemed to be adolescents. The line ambled along. Finally I reached the entrance. As I went in, I asked the man who was counting how many had come through. He said 13,768 so far, and the number would double before the day ended.

Inside, hundreds of people were milling about. It was quiet except for soft sobs and sniffing. Entering the huge main room I saw panels 6' by 3' laid out on the floor as far as the eye could see. One could walk down canvas aisles between the large sections and see the quilt pieces close up. The size of the project made unmistakably clear the enormity of the tragedy. Each panel represented a person killed by AIDS, yet only 10 percent of the people who have died of AIDS were represented in the quilt at this time. It was a bit like visiting a war memorial cemetery, except that instead of stones marking the lives of fallen warriors, pieces of soft fabric commemorated the lives lost.

I looked for Dennis's name among the list of people memorialized by quilt panels, and he wasn't there. I felt bad about that. Why hadn't Mark done one? Why hadn't I? Joe Robertson wasn't there either, but I know he died last fall. Occasionally I saw a panel naming a woman.

The quilt was conceived of by Cleve Jones, a long-time Bay Area activist. It first gained public attention at the big march on Washington in the fall of 1987 when 500,000 gay and lesbian people marched. It was an historic time. The purpose of the march was to focus public attention on the need for AIDS research and treatment funding, as well as to call attention to gay rights issues.

Brightly colored, the quilt pieces portray lives full of vitality and youth. They are created out of levis, sequins, shiny silver mylar, zippers, glass beads, ribbon, feathers, glitter, and everyday objects. They all carry messages of love. One carefully sewn panel included a photo of a pet cat and a pair of scissors, showing that he used to cut hair. Over and over people had indicated the dates of the person's life. I found myself subtracting 1957 from 1987—thirty years old. That's not old enough to die—he was younger than me! What a shallow pool of time these men played in.

Some panels were sewn from clothing the person wore. Sometimes photographs were sewn into the fabric. Some were very skillfully presented; others had been created with more love than skill. Most were sewn, but some were painted, made with felt pens, or silk screened. In one, the man's name was spelled out in his neck ties. The persons who sewed or assembled them chose symbols that had been key elements of their loved one's life. I saw lots of American flags, rainbows, military symbols, and objects indicating the person's profession. Often the names of the quiltmakers were hidden away in a corner. "Love, Mom and Dad." Occasionally there was a message: "Please: more prayers, more funding." Another: "The best Daddy in the world—died of AIDS in March 1987. I love you forever Daddy." And: "Oh, he did like to dress up!" One I particularly puzzled over had a name and the note, "Only lived one month— who killed him?"

Some quilt pieces were not for individuals. Nurses from one hospital made a quilt in memory of all the AIDS patients they had cared for. Some were anonymous: "I have decorated this banner to honor my brother. Our parents did not want his name used publicly. The omission of his name represents the fear of oppression that AIDS victims and their families feel." Another quilt was made "For those who have died alone."

Each panel told its own story, reflecting the humanity, interests, and personality of the person who had died. This was not a story of victims; it was a story of suffering, courage, fear, anger, and love. One could really get a sense of vibrant, vital people who had laughed, worked, played, and lived full and passionate lives. And in a larger sense, this quilt conveyed a picture of a people wrestling with an epidemic. Those who sewed the panels, those who have had to grapple with the reality of AIDS in themselves or loved ones, all came together in the quilt. This virus is a horrible killer, a tragedy that is happening in my time.

Here and there on a panel would be a fresh daisy, a bunch of flowers, or a little Christmas tree. Obviously someone who had loved the person had brought these things. Occasionally I would come upon a person kneeling or sitting at a panel as if they had been there for a long time. Maybe they just wished to spend the day with their lost friend. As people walked around and met others they knew, they would hug quietly and talk softly together. This was a sacred place and a holy experience, and I was deeply moved by it. I was glad these people have not gone unremembered, especially at this season.

A lot of people have been taken from us by this epidemic. These quilt panels represent only a small percentage of them. Where is the research money to stop the deaths?

I met an old friend and we hugged closely. My face was damp from very quiet tears of acknowledgment of a sad and powerful reality that is happening in my time, largely in my city, and to my generation.

February 1988—June said at breakfast that AIDS is the leading killer of women in New York City between the ages of 21 and 35. I was stunned. It's happening to my group too? How can that be? I guess it is because of IV drug use. From my work in Sixth Street Park, I know that often people who are stuck in drugs are deeply sensitive people who are in great pain. It is hard to admit that I have less sympathy for a person who is doing something that is individually and socially dangerous than I do for another person who might get the virus.

June and I are both worried about Alfredo, a gay man who works in the New York office who is terrified of getting AIDS. An old friend of his came to visit six months ago. Alfredo intimated that they had sex, and several weeks later the friend called and said that he had known at the time that he has AIDS. Is that murder? What suspicion must be riddling the gay world! How awful! Maybe there should be a law that anyone who knows that they are HIV positive and engages in unprotected sex without warning the other person should be guilty of a crime similar to murder.

I heard the other day about a man who was HIV positive who is a prostitute and refuses to stop his work. They have decided to arrest him to keep him off the streets. Boy. We are going to need a whole new set of laws and ethics codes to deal with this epidemic. How should society treat people who are HIV positive and refuse to act responsibly? What about quarantining them? That is a really tough question. Although they have rights, their lack of responsibility makes them a real threat, and we have to protect ourselves from them. Some people have suggested making them wear an electronic monitor so that if their blood pressure rises, the police are alerted. That sounds incredibly cruel and Brave-New-World-ish, doesn't it?

Of course the real answer lies in a new sense of responsibility on the part of everybody to protect themselves. We are all going to have to change. No more spontaneous sex; rather, we'll have to wait to be sure our test result is negative, and practice safe sex in the meantime.

One time when I was talking about nuclear issues with high school kids, one of them expressed anger at my generation for ruining sex for their generation. I am glad I lived during the days of free and unfearful sex. Although as a woman there was always the fear of pregnancy, that fear was connected to the possibility of another life springing from the sexual act. This new fear is connected to the possibility of death. So some of the ground gained in my generation about sex being fun and good may be lost in this epidemic. Damn.

March 1988—I saw a story on TV about a man with AIDS who volunteers in a kindergarten in the Haight. When some of the parents learned that he has AIDS, they pulled their children out of the school.

How do we know that tomorrow we won't find that the disease can be transmitted nonsexually? This disease is so young that very little is known about it. But at this point, medical authorities seem sure that it can be spread only via blood and body fluids. The parents who kept their kids in school had researched the known facts and felt that these children were safe.

It isn't hard to understand ignorance in this time, but it is hard to accept it. The kids interviewed love the man and very much value him playing and building things with them. And he just wants to put his life's energy into a useful activity—one that has something to do with a future he probably won't see.

From time to time now I read of a child who is excluded from a school because he or she has AIDS. The parents of the other children in the school band together to demand that the child be dismissed and forced to learn at home. But those children need to be around other kids. They aren't sick; they simply have a virus inside of them.

The parents' main fear is that the HIV-infected child will bite another child, break the skin, and thereby infect the second child. Doctors say it is very unlikely that the concentration of the virus in the saliva would be high enough to infect a child, even if the skin did break (which is unusual—how many times do kids bite other kids that hard anyway?). The problem, of course, is that when you say to a kid, "Don't bite other kids," you increase the odds that the kid will bite!

One concern that parents never discuss in articles or on television is their fear of children's sexual play. Children have always played "doctor" and probably always will, but they don't play overt sex games in classrooms. So kids with AIDS pose no greater danger in that regard. At home parents can supervise their children when they play with HIV-positive kids. I suppose some precautions are necessary, but children with AIDS should be allowed to live as normal a life as possible.

April 30, 1988—I decided to take the AIDS test and so today was the day. My sexual juices have been flowing these days and if these feelings lead me to want to "go vaginal" I want to do it responsibly. My doctor pressured me to get the test several months ago. At that time I had said to her, "Okay, let's do it right now," in a spontaneous act of bravado. But my doc said there was no way she could protect my privacy in this public hospital. She urged me to go to a public health center where testing was anonymous. I reassured her that the chance that I would be positive was really very small.

Yesterday I called the testing center and they had an appointment open for today. That surprised me. I thought they would have a long waiting list.

On my way to the testing site, I thought, "I really don't think I have AIDS. I don't even get colds, so I think my immune system is in great shape." If I were going to get AIDS from that one time of intercourse with Dennis about fifteen years ago, I would probably have it already. The only problem is that I took blood transfusions from the San Francisco blood supply nine years ago. One hospitalization alone with endometritis resulted in five transfusions.

I went into the waiting room. Sitting there were six men quietly staring straight ahead. No one was accompanied by friends. Absolutely nothing was said between any of us as we were ushered in to see the video—a pretty good one, actually. The person from the testing center came in to talk to us and answer our questions. He really spooked me. He paced in front of the room, never making eye contact with us. His ten-minute lecture was geared toward men and had very little information about women. When he asked if there were questions, in that environment I could not bring myself to ask any. Here I was, not even really afraid about the test—yet still intimidated by this environment of fear. How much harder it must be for the men being tested.

Then we went into the nurse one at a time. She tried to be friendly as she drew blood, but by now I don't think anyone was reachable. I walked out into the sun, glad to escape.

May 8, 1988—It has been an easy and good week. I have not thought about the test or felt any particular stress all week. But when I went to church, sitting with so many gay men and probably hearing the word "AIDS" a few times just in the flow of the service, I decided that I should find a pamphlet about what to think about before you get the results of the test. I looked in the pamphlet rack—nothing. I went up to the AIDS minister—yes, in my church and in some other San Francisco churches, there is a special ministry for AIDS patients. Carlene looked for a pamphlet and asked about the person needing it, assuming I was getting it for someone else. Finally I copped to the fact that I was the one who had taken the test, and I was looking for a pamphlet to guide myself. She seemed surprised.

I knew returning to the testing center could be tense, just from the terrifying experience of taking the test in that environment. I wanted to think about the issues involved in getting the results. And of course there is always the nagging fear about the outside chance that I could be positive. Talking about it reminded me how afraid of a positive test I really am.

I mostly focused on the problems I have with the medical world as I have no insurance. I have tried very hard—and so have many of my friends—to get health insurance. The fact that I am fat rules me out, the health insurance consultant says. What a system we have! This is a continuing problem whether or not I have AIDS. I talked about how angry I feel about the position my friends would be in if I were hospitalized with something really serious.

Maybe I should go to Sweden if I get sick. That's what my friend Michael thinks. Or maybe emigrate to Canada. The U.S. and South Africa are the only industrialized nations without some form of health insurance for all citizens. It really pisses me off how much suffering is caused by this backward attitude. One of the blessings of AIDS may well be that our present health system will go broke with the bill for this epidemic, moving us into some form of nationalized health care.

I don't know any women with AIDS so I guess I also think I am gender-immune. They say our vaginas are thicker than the walls of men's asses. So the virus is less likely to get into our systems. It's the only instance I have heard of where our reproductive system makes us less vulnerable than men.

After talking with Carlene I feel a little more aware of some of my hidden feelings about the test. I am sorry I have brought it up to the few people I have mentioned it to. Casually, almost flippantly, I have told five people who are not exactly the people I would have chosen if I had thought about it. Like David and Sharon from work. I told them just in line of what I had done that week. Sharon made me promise to tell her when I got the results. I couldn't possibly tell them if I did get a positive test.

Carlene offered to go with me to get my results, but I felt too frozen to respond. I'll think about it later in the week.

Saturday, May 14, 1988—I guess this journal is going to take a turn I never expected. I felt nervous going to get my test results. A funny thing happened on my way to the clinic. I had wanted to stop at the gardening store and get a hose. As I pulled in to my parking space, I noticed a tank-like vehicle parked across the street. This seemed strange. One doesn't see many tanks on the streets of America. But just then four police cars converged on the street and circled the tank. I ignored the commotion and went in to get my hose. When I came out the police were cavorting around the tank, pretending they had captured it. They were having a very good time, shouting and posing for pictures. Evidently this tank was in the neighborhood for a movie. I had never seen policemen carrying on like that on duty, and I wondered if we should be paying them to have so much fun. Isn't it funny the details you remember when sustaining a shock?

So when I arrived at the clinic, I was somewhat distracted by this event. The health educator saw me right away. She asked if wanted to talk about anything before she gave me my results. I said no, hoping she was not going to keep me over this cauldron of suspense for very long.

She said the results were "positive."

For a moment I was confused. What did "positive" mean? Did she mean it is a positive thing that I am AIDS-free? She read my mind. "It means you have the AIDS antibodies in your body," she said. "I want you to see for yourself." She blocked off the other results on her computer printout and instructed me to match up my number with the number on the list. "Here are the four tests they did with your blood," she continued. "The results are pretty conclusive."

I looked at her, then at the floor. I wanted to get out of there fast. What was I to do now? Now I wished there was someone waiting for me outside, someone into whose arms I could collapse. I felt trapped.

Here was this nice person who didn't know me from Adam, and I was completely exposed with her. And I didn't know what to do or say.

After a few minutes of staring silence, tears came to my eyes, and the stillness was broken by her touching my arm and offering Kleenex. I didn't cry hard. The tears just rolled down my face. "What shall I do?" I asked helplessly.

The whole thing is a blur now, but I think she said I should talk to lovers or former lovers. She asked if I took drugs. I said no. She was very interested in how I thought I had contracted the virus. I told her I was sure it was blood transfusions.

She drew a line on a piece of paper. She said all the people with positive tests are somewhere on this line. On the right side she wrote "AIDS" and in the middle, "ARC." On the left side she wrote "0" followed by "smt." Then she said that "0 smt" was me. I had never heard of the "0 smt" disease so I was even more confused than before. I can't begin to tell you how caught I was in the tumbling of an undercurrent of a large wave that had suddenly snatched me from the world of okay-ness. All the while she was talking about something and I was supposed to be paying attention. Finally I asked her what "0 smt" meant, and she said "no symptoms." She asked if I had swollen glands. I touched my neck and said, "I don't think so." She got out of her chair and felt my neck. It was nice to be touched at that moment. She said "no swelling." That was nice confirmation.

All jumbled up in my mind is some discussion about sore throats and night sweats. She again strongly encouraged me to tell my sex partners. If I wanted, the health center would make the calls without giving my name. I said I could do it myself although I didn't want to. She also said that I should tear up my organ donor card. Now that I had this virus, no one would want my eyes, liver, or heart for a transplant. That made me especially sad.

She got me talking about my work. I told her a little about it. We discussed the issue of secrecy which even now, a day and a half later, is terribly confusing for me. I asked her if I had to tell my doctor. She said no, but that it would help her treat me if she knew.

She said a very few support groups for women exist, but that I might not feel so comfortable in them because they were mainly for drug users. She said there were few services of any kind for women with AIDS, but suggested that I pick a few friends to talk it over with who could support me "in all the ways you will need support now." She told me that many people who receive negative test results experience survivor guilt because so many of their friends test positive. That didn't make me feel any better.

Somehow, blessedly, the conversation came to an end. It had been nearly an hour. I went home, unloaded the hose from the car and carried it back to the garden. Then I sat down next to the fig tree to think. I had planted this fig tree in the middle of my nuclear despair back in the early 1980s when I seriously wondered if we were going to blow ourselves up with nuclear weapons in the near future. Now it was a great comfort to see how tall and strong the tree was, and to remember how that despair had passed.

How long I was there I don't have any idea. After a while someone at the gate to the garden called out my name. It was Carlene, the AIDS minister from church. Rather automatically I told her to come in, although I knew I wasn't ready to talk. We sat silently until it became too cold to stay outdoors. I walked through the garden picking some food for her to take home with her.

Then Betsy came by and the three of us sat inside and talked. I don't remember much about what was said, except that I felt my emotions get damp twice. Once was when I told them about my sister having a baby that week and naming him after me. How special it was to know that she values me and wants my name carried in our family! There I was thinking about my own mortality, and the contrast of this little guy going into the future with my name was comforting.

Another moist moment was when Polly, my calico cat, came up to be close to me. I felt her love and acceptance. She has been with me through so much, and is a terrific comforter and friend.

Things were pretty full and pretty dark and still hard for me to sort out. One thing Carlene said several times in the course of the evening was that things would be changing now. There was no rush to do anything now, she said, because things would be changing. I didn't understand what she meant, and I didn't find it at all comforting. But I think it was a good thing to say. Betsy also said maybe it was better that I didn't have health insurance or a lover, since so many people lose those upon becoming HIV+ anyway. That didn't help much either, but it was an interesting perspective.

Betsy stayed the night. I made the bed for her in the office, but then asked if she could just hold me for a while. She said she would try to sleep in the bed with me. I assured her that my snoring would keep her awake and she should feel free to sleep in the other room. When she held me in her arms, the physical connection so contradicted my loneliness that in that moment I felt safe. I could share my fear in a deeper and easier way. We talked for a long time. I asked her to sing a song she had written about "not letting the darkness eat up the light." Then I turned on the TV and watched first a Jack Benny rerun, then Saturday Night Live. I lay on my stomach, my traditional way of sleeping, and Betsy lightly rubbed my back until I dozed off. For the moment, I felt safe and fine.

I awoke shaky and fearful in the night and had a hard time falling asleep again. So many questions and feelings were flashing through me. For instance, should I institute new hygienic practices like no kissing on the mouth (to protect myself as well as others)? Should I tell the people I have slept with in the last nine years? And what can I do to stay healthy? Who to tell and who not to tell has become a most important question on my mind. If I tell people at work, will they continue to let me work? Will people be afraid of me? What about my family? What should I do now? What's going to happen to me? Who will take care of me if I am sick?

I decided to tell no one for now. If David and Sharon asked me about the test results, I would tell them that I had missed my appointment because I wasn't sure that I wanted to learn the results of the test. That last part was true. Upon reflection, I wasn't sure that I wanted to know.

Sunday, May 15, The Next Day—In the morning I went to a workshop I had signed up to attend months ago. I couldn't bear to be with people, so I left after about an hour and went on a long walk. Later in the day, I called my family and was pleasant with them, not even hinting that anything was on my mind. The new baby, Jason Francis, was home and doing well.

I went to church in the evening feeling lonely and lost. As I looked around I knew that a lot of the men sitting would have answers to many of my new questions. "They will know where I can learn how to stay healthy, where to get into a support group to help me think through things," I told myself. "But I don't know any of these men well enough to ask them. Possibly some of the women know the men better than I and could help me. Also I know one of the women worked with AIDS patients in the prison system. Surely she would be able to point me in a direction to get some health information and advice." I thought I would just talk to four of the older women with whom I had felt some connection, asking for their help.

After the service I asked Karen if she and her partner Gail had a few minutes. She said, "No, we have to run some dishes out to San Leandro." Feeling hurt and unable to figure out the relative importance of dishes going to San Leandro as compared with my need for help at that moment, I wandered around.

Sylvia came over and hugged me and asked how the test had turned out. I couldn't find any words to tell her. Of course she guessed what that meant. She held onto me and started crying. I finally said, "I can't do this here." Feeling embarrassed and exposed, I pulled away as quickly as possible.

Then I bumped into Gail, the partner of the woman who had the dishes from San Leandro. In response to her routine question, "How are you?"—I told her. Karen came up with a couple of others and I shared with them what was going on. Karen (blessedly) said right away, "I don't believe these tests." And you know, I realized there was a part of me that didn't either. I am so grateful to her for putting that right out. Maybe there was a mistake. Maybe I should take another test. Maybe I am not really HIV+.

And now it is morning, barely 40 hours since the fateful visit to the clinic. I've been writing this since early morning with no break for breakfast. A calm is currently reigning over my emotions. I am grateful to have this journal. I began it years ago to be put into an archive of this epidemic someday; but now it feels like a friend in whom I can confide as I try to sort out what's happening to me. Just writing this today has been great therapy. And I'm ready for lunch.

May 16, Monday—Gail suggested right away that we meet the next evening to talk. So we did. We went to a Mexican restaurant and ordered something I was barely able to eat, my appetite having not really fully returned. I had lots of questions. I asked her if I should scrub the toilet seat when I have company over. She said no—that was unnecessary and would be bad for me. She said it so clearly that I believed her. "You should not think of yourself as a plague, as a pariah, someone that people have to be protected from. This is a dangerous attitude for you and for people you are close to." Later she also said, "There are people who have had antibodies in their blood for ten years and still are healthy and symptom-free."

Feeling really good about my talk with Gail, I went off to my theater class. I participated fully, not with my mind half on something else.

A friend—one I had been attracted to a week ago—called today. I was shocked that this person, whom I would have loved to get a call from two days ago, was someone I now wanted to stay away from. He just called to see how I was. I kept the discussion on a light and impersonal level. Do I blame him because it was my attraction to him and our petting that inspired me to think that I had better get ready to be sexual, and that is why I got tested? Do I think he is simply too lightweight to handle this? Or do I not want anyone that close just now? Who knows? I hope I do someday.

May 17, Tuesday—After a night filled with nightmares and fitful sleep, waking once crying for something lost down a well, I awoke at 5:45. I felt momentarily calm, then fear and panic rushed in. I go back and forth like that a lot. It's kind of like this year's unpredictable weather: up and down, sunny and wet. It's like falling into a wilderness—wild things occasionally leap out at me unexpectedly from behind rocks.

I occasionally consult with a therapist about a situation in my family. In today's session, however, I could talk only about myself. There are some issues about suicide that I don't want to discuss with my friends. I cried in the session, thinking that I would miss myself if I died. It sounds kind of illogical but it was an honest sentiment. I am shocked at the shame I feel when I talk about this virus inside of me. Where did that come from? They tell us where the virus comes from, but this secondary infection—shame—where does that come from?

Several times during the day I have felt so crumpled and broken. It's like a roller coaster. Sylvia wrote a note wondering why I had not been able to share what I was going through with her. I responded:

> Dear Sylvia,
>   Thanks for the note. I guess I didn't tell you how comforting it was to talk about computers the other night. I can't talk openly about deep frightening things while exposed in the church or while eating dinner in a restaurant. Also, by Sunday night I was tired of living in my feelings. I needed to leave AIDS and just be me for a while. I will have to play this by ear until I get a better handle on it, as it is all so new—a fresh and confusing wound. There is no rush—I am doing one thing a day on it now, and trying to keep calm. Please be patient with me. I don't know how to do this yet.
>   Sincerely,
>
>   Fran Peavey

Wednesday—Woke up after a very bad night's sleep. Had planned breakfast with two friends who I thought might have useful information about AIDS. I told them I had a friend who had just gotten a positive HIV test, and I was trying to help her. Arthur said that there are not many services for women. I am looking for a women's support group or just someone I can talk to who knows that women too can get this disease.

I talked to my close friend Kathleen. At first I could barely bring myself to say anything to her at all. A few tears came occasionally as I talked about my nephew being named after me, but the dam really broke loose when I said I was going to need her help now. She drew me close and I held onto her tightly as I sobbed. She was pretty emotional too.

It is hard to remember how dependent we are upon the help of others, and this knowledge is buried in turds of pain.

Thursday—This morning I went over to talk with one of the women,

Kathy, in my little group of four at church. She works with men in Vacaville prison who have AIDS. It's really hard to imagine being in prison with all this going on inside. She says that the men are ostracized in prison by both inmates and prison personnel. This is very hard on them. The prisons are having a tough time figuring out what to do with HIV+ people. She is teaching visualization techniques to the prisoners. It is so fine to think of someone reaching out and teaching these people who are trapped in two prisons—a legal one and one created by a virus. Her visualizations are creating ways for them to escape feeling so totally imprisoned by reaching for the resources without barriers, available to them through their own minds. She teaches me too.

I have actually been considering doing something I thought I would never do—talk to the people in my company about this news. Things do change minute to minute.

Also, today I heard my voice saying for the fortieth time that I can't go to these HIV+ support groups which are made up only of men. I don't like to hear my voice saying "I can't" very often. It does not build a habit of courage or a positive self-concept. Since I have not been able to find a mixed or women's support group, I guess I may have to learn how to be the only woman in an all men's group.

So I went to a group today. When they asked why I had come, I said that I just wanted to see if I could come to a group like this. Carlene ran the group, so of course she knew why I was there, but I wasn't ready to reveal my HIV+ status to a group of people I didn't know. What I found out from going to this is that there are fine people in the group, but I feel out of place. In my work life, I am often in meetings where I am the only woman; in such situations I feel similar discomfort. I hate having a disease that is known primarily as a man's disease.

Friday—There is so much research I need to do now. Fortunately, some friends are doing some of it for me. For instance, a friend has finally found a support group for HIV+ women. Another is looking into vitamins which will build my immune system.

One Week after Test Results—On Saturday afternoon I found myself getting anxious and agitated. I was working in the house writing a report. I stopped and thought, "It's been one week now." So, almost automatically, I went to the garden and sat by the fig tree to review the week. One thing was obvious: It had been a rough week! I had gotten little real work done. I went through some pretty difficult places thinking about running away, about the day coming (sometime) when I might be sick or die. I cried hard, sitting in the warm sun. I cried for myself, for the shame and confusion I feel, and for how unfair it is for me to have to deal with this when I am busy with other things. But I also thought about the real victories this week. I have been able to talk with a few people, and they have been kind.

Another victory is the research I have been doing. I am beginning to figure out where the resources are in this community for health information, as well as an underground "Buyers Club" where one can purchase medicines not allowed on the market. There is a meeting once a month where the most up-to-date information is discussed, as well as a computer teleconference for day-by-day discoveries. I am really amazed at the extent and variety of the infrastructure responding to this epidemic.

In my effort to understand what has happened to me, I came up with this statement: A civic-minded man, probably gay, gave blood at a time when the technology could not distinguish infected blood from noninfected blood. I was given that blood by a doctor who was trying to keep me from bleeding to death. And now I have been told that there are antibodies to the AIDS virus in my blood. My body has done a very smart thing by making those antibodies. It shows that it is fighting the disease and probably winning. Go, body!!!

I talked to Carlene to check out this statement for accuracy. I was stunned when she said I still had the virus inside me. I asked incredulously, "You mean the virus is inside of me right now? Why don't my antibodies kill it?" She said it was living in my body right now. I said, "Where is it? What is it doing now?" She said it was all over, it was everywhere in my blood.

I felt devastated. This situation is too massive to understand. It's not like cancer where the problem is in one location. It's not like diabetes where the problem is sugar. The problem is omnipresent in something I need: blood.

Wednesday—This was a fruitful day. I wrote on India early in the day. At work I had meetings all day. I was able to participate solidly and felt appreciated for my contributions. I was light and fun at various points during the day.

On Monday I had told David, a friend and colleague, about my test results. Actually he and Sharon had guessed that the test was positive. On Wednesday David accompanied me to a lecture on "Women and AIDS." This had to be one of the most awful experiences of my life. A very clinical, statistically minded speaker stood up and talked about what AIDS does to the body, and what the disease is like. She said that women who are HIV+ (she used the word I don't like the sound of, "seropositive") are different from men who are "seropositive." On the average, women tell only two or three people. I don't know why we would be more secretive than men. Maybe it is because for women, AIDS is not yet a reality and we don't know how to respond to it. When a gay man in the Castro learns that he is HIV+, his friends know what to do and where to send him for the support and information he will need; they also know how to stay calm in the midst of his terror. An HIV+ woman is on her own. She has to start from the ground up, educating her friends, finding resources which will allow her to make good health decisions. It's tough sledding between the fear and denial of friends who are unfamiliar with the virus. They don't really know what to do and how to be helpful.

The speaker had all the statistics, and she handed copies out to us. One was the latest scoop on how many people had tested positive for the virus as of two weeks ago. It felt spooky to see myself as a statistic, since that was the exact week I had gotten my results. There I was, tallied anonymously on the paper—part of the epidemic.

But what really got me was when she said something about how having the HIV virus in your body may be enough to affect your mind. Short-term memory may deteriorate. And another "cheery" statistic: 75 percent of the people with HIV get AIDS and die.

After fifteen minutes, I wanted to get out of there. I didn't think I should be listening to this. It was too hard. I felt it was dangerous to my health. But I knew if I left, people would think I had AIDS. So I would have to tough it out. To think that my brain could be affected right now—hey, this is serious! I felt devastated. Tears welled up in me as I walked out. When we got to the car I couldn't hold back the flood anymore. The wave of hopelessness and emotion poured out of me. I felt utterly flattened by emotions. This was a threat to my most vulnerable place: my thinking, my mind. David held me as I sobbed in the car.

A Few Days Later—Gail had suggested I visit a doctor she knows with lots of experience with AIDS, so I made an appointment with Lisa. Lisa's office is on Castro Street (no wonder she has lots of AIDS patients). I had decided to use a pseudonym for today's visit.

Lisa, the doc, immediately struck me as an energetic, confident woman with a relaxed sense of humor. Right away she asked me how I was doing with the news of being HIV+. Then she asked about my support system. She looked at my tongue, felt my neck, listened to my heart—the usual things. She said I was fine. She started to write out a prescription for a T-cell count using the pseudonym I had given her, but I stopped her and told her it was an alias.

She asked why I had given another name, and I felt a little self-conscious but said that I didn't know about her files. I told her that I can't help thinking that there may come a day when this society becomes so frightened of the virus inside of us that they want to round us up. If society should turn ugly on the people who carry this virus, her office in the Castro would be one of the first places they would go to find out who was HIV+. She said she understood; many of her patients used a pseudonym.

I told her I was unsure whether it would be safe to talk to my own doctor at General Hospital. Could she call my doctor and ask whether she continues to see patients who are HIV+? Fortunately, Lisa had done her training at General and knew my doctor. She said she had no hesitation—Mimi would not dismiss me. I still feel worried about it, but I guess I just have to have some trust.

I asked her what symptoms I should watch for now that I know about the virus. She said she could tell me, but only if I would promise not to worry constantly about the symptoms. That made me hesitate. I said, "No, I would worry. You'd probably better not tell me." She replied that, in general, anything we should worry about I would worry about anyway, because it would be so noticeable. Mainly I should watch for fevers over 101 degrees and difficulty in breathing. She encouraged me to keep my stress down, talk to my friends, and practice safe sex. She also said that the study about HIV affecting one's short-term memory early in the infection was poorly done and that I shouldn't pay too much attention to it. We will see how the T-cell count goes.

A Week Later—It has been a while since I wrote. A lot has changed in my ideas about myself and my social context. In this time I have had my first bout with a fever. I hadn't slept for four or five nights and was exhausted. On Sunday I awoke with an ear infection which got progressively worse until by afternoon I could not escape the notion that I was sick. I had to cancel a river float trip that I had really looked forward to, and instead stay in bed. But worse, I had a fever. I know this sounds strange, but my thermometer only measures to 100 degrees. Since I am rarely sick, I had never noticed that it was a conception thermometer and not a regular thermometer. When the mercury topped out at 100, I freaked out. The doctor had said that if I had fevers around 101 degrees, I should let her know. Panic flooded me.

I kept telling myself that I have had ear infections many times in the past. Just because I was now worried about my immune system, I shouldn't freak out about every symptom being the beginning of the end. Still, I remembered hearing on the radio of a guy who died of an ear infection rather than go to a doctor and hear that he had AIDS.

Exposed To Vulnerability

I hate it when others see
and force me to see too
that self I am
stripped of the dignity I have mindlessly developed

and all the artifices I have stolen from civilization
to make myself presentable.
I hate it when my body takes over control
trembling
sobbing
tearing
vomiting.

That anyone should see me in that way
humiliates me
yet draws me so close
and so comforts the wildness inside.

People often say "Show me your vulnerable side."
Ah, to be able to throw up at will.

Two Weeks Later—Things I've Learned at the Feet of the AIDS Virus:

- I change more rapidly than I ever could have imagined. Previously I could not conceive of talking to the people I work with in the Internews company. Absolutely not, I thought—they wouldn't let me continue to do my work if they knew. After one week of suffering silently in their presence with my new situation, feeling isolated and separate, I told them one by one—and they were fine about it. Over and over they asked, "How will your life change now?" A very good question.
- People really are kind, even when confused, frightened, and stunned. In spite of all my fears about talking to people close to me, 100 percent of them (about 10 at this point) have shown me gentleness and kindness—the very opposite of the rejection I feared from them.
- People are more willing to help when they know specifically what kind of assistance would be the most appreciated. I have been having trouble sleeping in this period (a very rare problem in my life). Finally I asked some friends if I could come and sleep at their house. I fell asleep immediately, and when I awoke I noticed they had left their door open as if to say, "If you get scared in the night,

we are here." It was so comforting that I dozed right back off.

- A luxury which many people do not appreciate is that of walking around without a concern for how much time one has left, and with few worries about the quality of life on the road to that death. Many people share this lack of security with people who are HIV+. People who are old, people who are hungry, people in physical pain, people in politically unstable regions, people in wars...in fact, most of the people in the world, by my calculations, share these worries. So I have left the carefree, mindless minority to join the alert, precious majority who know about the limits of life, who are constantly aware of the suffering that is basic to life, and who carry close to themselves the warm appreciation of being alive today.

- Telling people you are HIV+ isn't as hard as one might think. In general, I have tried to tell people on the phone so they could have time to get it together with themselves before I saw them again. Another helpful thing is letting them know who else in our friendship circle knows about it, so they can talk together and support each other. Two people are usually smarter than one in this area.

- One doesn't always need to be completely truthful. In several instances where people asked why I wasn't my usual playful self, I didn't feel I wanted to share the reason with them. So I simply said, "I've had some upsetting news in my family." This was true enough and it got me out of an embarrassing situation.

- I need to spend a little time each day moving myself forward on this situation, but I also have to be sensitive to my limits. I have allotted one hour a day now to researching how to stay healthy and thinking about what to do. The rest of the day I do my work and play.

- Often people talk about AIDS and don't know what they are talking about or who they are talking to.

- Here are a few things I think are especially important to remember: (a) Nothing is wrong with my body. All HIV+ means is that my body has met the virus and has developed antibodies. People can live a long time with those antibodies fighting the virus. (b) HIV+ is not a death sentence. It reminds us that we will die someday and maybe sooner than later, but probably not today—unless we are hit by a truck (as my doctor says).

- It stuns the human spirit to have news like, "You're HIV positive" said about the body which is the spirit's home. It may take a while to feel like your old self. You have to consider the possibility that you may never be your same familiar self again—and that may be really good for you.

June 2, 1988—I had a regularly scheduled visit with my doctor, so I determined that at that visit I should discuss with her my HIV+ news and how that affected our relationship. She is a rather formal person, preferring to call me Ms. Peavey although I consistently call her Mimi. She works in a public hospital and is one of the teaching physicians. She carries lots of responsibilities, although she doesn't act officious or pompous.

I talked a little about the stomach pains I had been having for over a year. She wondered if it was some parasite which we had not been able to find in the traditional ways.

Finally I took a big breath and said that there was something I needed to discuss with her. Then I just blurted it out. Later I thought that this was sort of an unusual situation—usually the doctor is the one who tells the patient bad news and therefore has a chance to prepare for the experience. Here the tables were turned and she was totally unprepared. She seemed visibly stunned by the news. I remember she said in a very sincere way, "Oh, I am so sorry!"

Then she asked how I was doing with it. Mimi is a great one for checklists and, after a little discussion about how I don't need to feel ashamed for having this problem, I could almost see her open a mental file called "HIV+ checklist." She asked why I had taken the test, forgetting that we had discussed it months before and that she had strongly urged me to take it. She said I should tell some friends and learn to talk with them about what is going on inside of me about this. "Isolation is the real killer in this thing," she said. I said I was doing pretty well with that, although I found it much easier to talk with people who knew about AIDS than with my long-time friends who were pretty AIDS-illiterate and fearful. She asked about telling sexual partners and about new safe sex habits. When I stood to leave I remember she gave me a little hug. I was not prepared for this unusual connection with her—I hardly knew what to do.

June 10, 1988—The nurse at the testing clinic who told me I was HIV+ had stressed that I should talk to people I had had sex with, and let them know that they might also be infected. She was quite insistent about this, and I understand why there is a need to take this responsibility seriously. Communicating to people that they might be at risk is, of course, a key in stopping the spread of the epidemic. In my support group (I joined a support group for HIV positive women a couple of days ago), a lot is said about telling ex- or present lovers. I knew it would not be easy. I dreaded it, in fact. I figure that since the men I have loved in the past nine years have always used condoms for birth control, they would be safe. The women I have loved, on the other hand, might be a different story.

I called Karla, the person I was most recently involved with, and asked if we could get together. I said I just wanted to talk. Since things were still quite raw between us, it did not seem unusual to get together to sort out our feelings and upsets with each other.

I met her early one morning. She wanted to go to a breakfast place. I said that I really didn't feel like talking in a restaurant—could we just sit in the car for a bit? "Sure," she said.

The news rolled out relatively easily. "I have some difficult news: I'm HIV positive," I said. I told her the likelihood that she was infected was extremely small—there have only been two cases of woman-to-woman transmission, and researchers are dubious about one of the cases. She seemed not so afraid for herself, but more upset about me and what this would mean in my life. I, of course, was afraid she would be mad at me. Our sex life and activities had been fraught with difficulty and crossed signals, and now to have this deadly threat associated with sex seemed to add insult to an already quite high pile of hurt. I was aware of a trembling deep in my backbone as I talked with her. It was not a long talk; I was not able to go into much depth because I was so frightened. She said she would take the test and practice safe sex until she knew her status.

She asked if I wanted breakfast now, but I was not the least bit hungry. So I drove off, leaving her on the curb to get breakfast alone. I drove around the corner, stopped the car, and broke down in tears. I had been so frightened she would be really angry and harsh with me, and I was scared I had hurt her by loving her.

June 11, 1988—A number of people associated with my work suggested that I call Bob and talk over my situation. His response was at first sympathetic; then he turned comic with, "Fran, you'll do anything to lose weight, won't you?"

I appreciated his humor about this. There hasn't been enough lightness about this pickle I find myself in.

June 15, 1988—At a party a friend who does not know my situation said she had been to a really wonderful retreat. "There was one person dying of AIDS—Richard." Once again I hear dying equated with AIDS. In my most patient, and perhaps somewhat paternalistic way, I said, "I think Richard would be insulted if he knew you thought of him as dying just now. He gets up in the morning and goes to work, socializes, and has fun. He has quite a full life. Just now it seems to me that he is living with AIDS. I think it is oppressive to have that dying-expectation surrounding him. It assumes an end which I am not sure Richard assumes just now. He is fighting for his life now. When he is in the bed taking his last breaths, that is the time to say he is dying."

I am tired of the AIDS-equals-death equation. And it is not

necessarily accurate. Riley has had the virus inside of him for nine years, and he is still doing great. There are many deaths, but it is not automatic—that is important to remember.

June 16, 1988—I was having company over and was slicing some vegetables when I cut my finger a little. I freaked out. How do I get the virus off the cutting board? And off the knife? And how do I make sure that it is not on the zucchini? What if the virus jumps out of the blood and starts running around?

At that exact moment, Sarah, a friend from Boston, called. With no thought for secrecy or anything, I gave her a full load of my concerns. Talking to her calmed me. I remembered that I would be cooking these vegetables anyway, so that would kill whatever might be there even though I had thrown away any vegetables I suspected of being tainted by my blood. And of course, this virus can't run around.

Also today I met another woman in my social circle who is HIV+. Kim and Ev heard from another friend that a mutual friend had AIDS. It took quite a bit of jockeying to get us connected since each friend had been pledged to secrecy, but finally we talked. It was interesting and she had lots of new-age theory, philosophy, and medical advice to share.

One thing she said really worried me. She said she had not been able to play with her friends who were children because she was afraid of giving them AIDS or of them being afraid of her giving them AIDS. She doesn't want to share her secret with their parents and let them decide what they want for their children, so she just avoids the children. She really misses these contacts. I tried to tell her that I thought it was unnecessary for her to deny herself: Why does she assume such ignorance on the part of her friends? But I understand the dynamic. It's a function of the secrecy. It is assumed as a part of a trusting relationship that if I am going to do something that I feel safe about doing, but which you might not feel safe about, then we will come to a mutual decision about how to proceed. But when secrecy is at play, then the basis of trust is violated.

When I came home, I called the AIDS hotline. They said I can play safely with children.

June 17—One of the ways to keep score in the AIDS ballgame is through T-cell counts. A T-cell count can tell you how active the virus is in your body. No standard has been determined exactly, but when the count gets down around 400 or 500 they know that the virus is acting up. Some people I have heard about have T-cell counts of 5 and are still walking around and working every day. But that means that there are very few T-cells to fight any infections that come along.

I sometimes wish that I had never taken the HIV test at all. My life is permanently changed now, and that sometimes overwhelms me. I don't like to think that I may never kiss deeply again. I like to think that problems can "be fixed," that there is a surgery that could be done or a treatment which could make things better. That isn't what is happening with this virus just now. Waves of anxiety come over me about this time-bomb inside of me. I feel silly because they are unrelated to anything except the news that I am HIV positive. I feel fine and my sense of my body is that it is fine too. But I have these periods of several hours' duration, when I feel terror at not knowing how things are going inside and what could happen.

June 18—I had an evening meeting with Jill last night. After we had done the bulk of our business, she asked me—as if she had been thinking about it for awhile—what was the story about me and kissing? She had noticed that I was reluctant to share Calistoga water at a concert we attended with a bunch of other people, and that I had been shy about casual mouth kissing recently.

I just haven't figured out what to do about kissing. I feel uneasy about doing things around the mouth until I get the research and find out more about it. I have been so busy trying to learn how to preserve my own life and what to do next, as well as just getting over the shock. I feel as though I have been knocked down and am not yet able to get up. And on top of everything else I have to think about kissing? Give me a break! It doesn't help that in order to figure out about things like kissing and sharing apples, I have to turn to government statistics. I, who have a life-long habit of distrusting what the government says. And who wouldn't? This same government that lied to me about Three Mile Island, Vietnam, and Nicaragua is going to give me information about kissing and expect that I should believe it? What is my option?

Jill asked me, "Does this mean that you won't kiss if you fall in love with someone?" I felt such an openness to the way she asked it that I surprised myself with the openness of my response. "I'll just have to see and work it out with the person. It will be a slow negotiation process—slower than usual. We will just have to figure it out together." This was a process statement rather than a tapped-down policy, and I kind of surprised myself with it. I am in a period of deep not-knowing right now. I am changing so rapidly every day that I often surprise myself—sometimes positively, as in this case, and sometimes negatively.

I'll call the AIDS hotline for information. Who would ever have thought that I would need to research kissing in my 46th year?

June 19—I was in a class at my church the other day. The teacher—

a large, middle-aged, generally jolly man—announced at the beginning of the class that he would be leaving us for about an hour in the middle to attend a funeral in another part of the building. "I'll be back in about an hour," he said, "probably a little red-eyed, but it will be okay." It seemed that he was quite accustomed to funerals at this point. It somehow made me think of battlefields; I have always had the sense that men at war take a bit of time out to take care of the dead, and then just get back to the business of fighting.

June 20—The AIDS hotline reports that one would have to exchange five gallons of saliva to get AIDS from kissing. Should I believe that? Anyway, I think I'll be a little easier about people who aim at my mouth for kisses. I have noticed a little "macho-kissing" from some people. "Let me prove to you that you are not untouchable with this AIDS virus inside of you," they seem to say. "I am not afraid, and I will prove it right now with this kiss."

I want to know how things will turn out, but I don't want to know if the news is bad. I am not so afraid of dying as I am of losing my mind and becoming a nothing. That is my greatest fear. From my talking with other HIV+ people I would say it is one of the most common fears. What I really cannot figure out is this: If you get dementia, will you remember that you had decided to do euthanasia, or do you forget everything? And do you notice that you are losing it or not? And are you humiliated by not having intelligence, or do you just slip into stupidness without self-consciousness?

At the Gay Freedom Parade I looked upon the faces of the guys in the 32 AIDS-related floats—out of over 86 floats in the entire parade—which went by me. I kept thinking that we need those guys solving some of the world's problems now, not losing it. Some time ago these were free-spirited, vital people, filled with life and energy. Now they are gaunt and tired-looking, with a stare that is hardly animated or energetic. Suddenly I realized that, without my noticing it, tears had been running down my face. A friend sitting next to me called my attention to it. All she said was, "You are really healthy, Fran." I was crying not only for myself right then, but for them and for our society and for what we are becoming. We don't seem to be able to stop all this dying, and it feels so helpless to face that. We have created a world of chemistry and radiation and pollution that our bodies are telling us we can no longer tolerate. Viruses are being born and killing us. What does it mean that a new virus has begun to strike human beings down? Something is happening in this world of ours, and it isn't good.

Sure, some of those tears were for me—I'm part of this. Now I sit watching this parade, not impacted enough to force me out of hiding and onto a float. I wondered about my own path with this virus, about my life and how it will go. What would I look like skinny—and gaunt? In my heart I felt new rumblings: these were my people.

I keep trying to get a picture of what is happening inside my body and to understand what has already happened. As well as I can comprehend it, the virus that entered my bloodstream is like poison inside of a bomb. That bomb could go off any time. My job is to care for that bomb as best as I can and not to pass it on to anyone else, either on purpose or unconsciously. The bomb is inside of me, and my body has done the best thing it could do: build antibodies (warriors to keep the virus from going off and lodging parts of itself in the soft parts of myself). This virus is devious. It only goes for the soft places, like the brain and mucus membrane around the sexual places.

June 22—Well, my first menstrual period since the test results came and went this week. Blood outside of my body. I looked at the blood on the pad. "This came from me and it could hurt someone else." This signifies a very real threat to my self-concept. I have always thought of myself as good. Sure, sometimes I have hurt people, but I have never thought of myself as having killing inside of me.

I was at a party where there was a hot tub. A friend who knows about my being HIV+, and also is aware of how much I love to relax in hot tubs, encouraged me to take a tub. I said that it was the first day of my period and I worried about blood leaking out and harming someone. At first she looked at me as if I were an old-fashioned woman unwilling to get wet during her period. Then she remembered and nodded. It seems likely that the hot water would kill these fragile buggers—but maybe not. Gosh, this is confusing! So much to research, so little reliable information.

The sands of reality are shifting all the time.

July 8—I called the AIDS hotline. They say that I can't give anyone the virus in a hot tub even if I am having my period. First the heat kills the virus, second the virus would be so diluted by the water that it would not be in sufficient concentration to hurt anyone. There has to be a bunch of viruses together to get anything going in another body. One little virus isn't enough.

This hotline is really a great idea. They are willing to give you the research on anything. They provide information in such detail that I believe them.

July 21—I finally got the time to go up to Humboldt County to visit David and Sharon. We really haven't seen each other to talk in depth since "I hit these skids," as I refer to my situation these days.

One thing Sharon shared with me helped me understand some of what my friends are going through. I have found it really difficult to talk with many of my friends because they seem so afraid and generally ignorant about the issues facing a person who is HIV positive. Sharon is a highly qualified nurse, the nursing director of the county hospice. She deals with AIDS people all the time. When she first heard of my status, she says she was stunned. More than that, she felt unable to talk with me about it. She said that now instead of AIDS affecting someone in her professional sphere, it was in her family—someone she cared deeply about. She felt totally unprepared to talk with me about her feelings or my feelings, or to share what she knew about AIDS. She was able to talk with me only after a visit to the county AIDS specialist in which she asked some very specific questions. I don't know what those questions were, but the key for me was that even with all her experience she felt inhibited in her relationship with me.

Now Sharon isn't like this. She is usually free to talk with any of us in our group about our health issues—she is sort of our unofficial health consultant. But here she was over her head—partly because of her fear, partly because of her love for me, and possibly partly because she has experience with AIDS. It is hard for her to think of that happening to me. Well, if it is that hard for her, with all of her background, it is easier for me to understand the behavior of my friends who have little information besides newspaper headlines about AIDS.

When I found out that I was HIV+, an invisible circle of friends began to form around me including a few old friends and some very new friends who were able to walk with me into a new reality. I am beginning to see why old friends are having such a tough time talking to me about these changes and finding out what they need to learn about HIV in order to move into the circle with me.

We also went on a really wonderful float trip down the Mad River. I think I am the happiest when I am floating down a river in an inner tube. That is heaven for me.

July 22, 1988—In my women's HIV+ support group we talk a lot about ethics and morals. The group consists of four women "regulars" besides me. One of the women got the virus from her husband, who died of AIDS before they had diagnosed his condition; one, an older woman (over 60), got it from a blood transfusion; and two women got it from sharing needles. Another two women left the group early on: one got the virus from drugs and was pregnant, and the other got it from her boyfriend who does IV drugs.

Our time together seems to be spent on three content areas: (1) Information about the disease, how it is spread and what we can do about it. We share resources, and the group leader gives little lectures about wellness and the philosophy of health. (2) Meditation and visualization techniques to reduce stress and promote wellness. (3) Discussion of the emotional issues relating to our being HIV+. Having this bomb inside us raises very important ethical issues. Do we have to tell our dental hygienist? Is there a way to "disclose" (HIV terminology) without telling her that you are positive? (Yes, they say: Gently ask her if she shouldn't be wearing gloves.)

Disclosure is a big question in our group. We are asked to imagine telling people about our virus status. For instance, I am trying to imagine telling my brother so that I can get the durable power of attorney paper filled out. The durable power of attorney is a paper my doctor wants which names the person authorized to make decisions on behalf of my body if my mind is not with it.

We also discuss the way we feel about our bodies. One woman last week said she felt stained and polluted. Everyone nodded.

But the thing that is the most interesting to me is when we talk about responsibility. I have been in lots of intellectual discussions about the relationship of the individual to the society, but never such vital discussions as these in our support group. Here alienation, ethics, and moral responsibility are not abstract concepts, but real day-to-day decisions. We have to grapple every day with our responsibility to others. We understand alienation because we live in a society where there is prejudice and ignorance. We must develop new senses of who we can be open with, who will hurt us, and how to deal with daily references to a situation which we are intimately connected to but not necessarily open about.

And we have to change our lives in ways that we don't necessarily like. Several of us say we could not possibly think of starting to date again. Would anyone want to love us?

Others share the rejection they have faced, how their partners deal with the restrictions of loving them. One woman's boyfriend cannot tell any of his friends about her being positive and about the compromises they make in their lives, because he knows he would be judged badly. Why couldn't he find a woman to love with whom he could have "real sex"? Another woman brought her boyfriend in to talk with the group leader about safe sex. He won't kiss her anymore, and that upsets her. The older woman will not talk to any of her friends because this disease carries such a stigma. All of her friends have "nice" diseases, like Parkinson's or cancer.

One woman told a story this week that moved me. She was sitting in a downtown outdoor café with her fellow workers on coffee break. Across the café a thin man entered, and her colleagues began talking about how they wished that the restaurant would not let AIDS guys in. She was feeling very hot inside about this discussion, because she knew the guy from a support group. Without saying anything to her colleagues, she just stood up, went over and gave him a hug, and then talked with him for a few minutes. Afterwards she went back to work by herself. She was really upset when she got to our group. Had she exposed herself by what she had done? Would they now want to get rid of her? She was angry at herself for not restraining herself, yet at the same time proud of her integrity.

I recently saw a couple of bumper stickers: "Anyone who thinks God gave AIDS as a punishment hasn't met our God." And another: "AIDS is a four-letter word."

July 22, 1988—I talked to Chris about some business today. In the discussion I mentioned that part of the reason for a particular decision I had made was my HIV status. His initial response was, "You're joking!" Then he said, "No, you're not joking. Who would be joking about this kind of a thing? You're the last person I would have suspected." Then he shared something I had always guessed: he was HIV+ too. Not only Chris, but also his lover, Brian. And Brian has been sick lately, he said. "I can't even imagine what I would do if Brian got very sick or...died." His voice lowered and his fears of separation and aloneness were evident. He told me that Brian is now on AZT and some other medicine I have never heard of. Brian's T-cell count is 225, while Chris's is in the 500s.

Chris mentioned something that meant a lot to me. He said that from all his experience (he has the names of thirty-five friends in his address book which he will not cross out because he would miss seeing at least the name, he says), no one goes through this alone. "Someone will be there. Not the person you might have expected, but someone who will care deeply and love you...and whom you will come to love too."

We parted promising to see each other very soon.

July 24, 1988—There are a lot of crazy things that occur to me daily now that I know the AIDS virus has made its home inside me. Tonight as I crossed the bridge and handed the toll taker my dollar bill, I thought how the toll taker would feel if he knew I was HIV+. Would he worry about infection? What if I spit on the bill? Would that worry him more? What if I rubbed it in my crotch? There is some part of me that enjoys thinking of "torturing" people who are afraid. Not that I would ever do those things, but I do think strange thoughts. These are ways of playing with the fear of others, rather than letting it get to me.

July 25, 1988—Today has been another rough day. I had a fever of almost 100 degrees and diarrhea, and no wind at all in my sails. I am totally exhausted. Yet I did not do much hard work yesterday and have no explanation for my exhaustion. I did little all day except some writing and some phone calls. I called my doctor to see what I should do. Upon finding she was not going to be in for two days, I was forced to talk to a nurse who pulled the story out of me and made an appointment for me at 1:30.

I took a nap before the appointment so that I could have the energy to go, but when I awoke I felt sicker and unmotivated to go to be hassled by the medical establishment. What would they tell me anyway? My body is fighting this virus, and today is one of those battles. I can feel the fight raging inside, and I feel more likely to win at home than sitting in some clinic with other sick people waiting forever to see someone I don't trust and being humiliated by questions from more people who don't know much about my condition. Better to stay home, rest here, and read a good book by Alice Walker about the human spirit and ancestors.

July 27—This week I finally decided to face head-on the issue of dementia. I have a hard time even remembering that word—and there is something appropriately peculiar about that! I wanted to do my initial exploration in a very private way. I did not want anyone who knew me to know that I was having these thoughts about my intelligence or the diminution of the same. People might start to have doubts about my abilities; this would be bad for my work, for my self-confidence, and for my health. People might think I was a hypochondriac, obsessing about things that are not happening yet. "After all, you are healthy," I heard my imaginary friends saying. "Don't worry until it happens." But of course if you wait until you are demented, how will you have a plan?

Ever since the talk on "Women and AIDS," this has been my big fear. It's one of the things which we infected people fear the most—probably even more than death. To be alive and not there—that's bad, especially when you are young and all your friends are still so much all there. My careers depend upon my smartness and quickness, and if those are no longer available to me, there must be other ways to make money.

I decided to do research on what abilities one might not lose to dementia. Then I planned to find books on occupational therapy and look up careers that would use talents likely to stay with me even if I began to lose it. I could start acquiring those skills now so that I would be ready. I wanted to do this research where nobody would know I was concerned about such things. I reasoned that I could do it in the East Bay where I am less known—where I have been in the newspaper less, taught fewer students, and performed less frequently.

I called the people at a certain AIDS institution with a consultant who could be a resource on dementia. They said that they could make an appointment for me, and what was my name? I wasn't prepared for that question.

"Do I have to tell you my name?"

"Yes, we need it for our files."

"Okay, I'll use ___ ."

For me the real challenge is remembering the false name I use in HIV-related appointments and answering to it. I really hate the feeling of deception that using this pseudonym creates, but I don't see a viable alternative right now.

I arrive for my appointment. "Please fill in these forms for us to get funding," says the person who greets me. "Name, address, phone number, social security number." Inside I think, "Oh, dear. What shall I do? I can't possibly make up and remember all this false information. Am I being paranoid, or is it possible that information about being HIV+ could be used against me? Maybe I should just give up and walk out of here. Why does this have to be so difficult?" I end up feeling the way I did as a child when I lied to my mother. But I give them some combination of truth and wild fiction. (I especially love making up social security numbers.)

I walk in to see the person I am consulting. He looks at me and tries to make me comfortable. He says, "I like your pants; they look very comfortable." "Thank you," I say, "I have them made in India where I work every year." And then he said—I swear he did it just this way even though it doesn't conform to my ideas of how people think or work—"Oh, are you Fran Peavey? I read your book. I loved it, every word." He recognized me from the picture in *Heart Politics*. Of course, it pleased me that he liked the book, and there is even some pleasure in being recognized. But how am I going to stay healthy if I can't even get information without jeopardizing my privacy? And what does it do to my body's sense of integrity to have this kind of lying about my identity going on? In some way this secrecy seems to compromise my health as much as the virus does.

Poem

Now I find I may walk through my life
   with the AIDS virus inside of me.
It was not gentle news
   but a hurricane which tumbled everything around within me.

I have no mother,
   no father to turn to for help with this.
I have no lover
   to cradle me in his or her arms and say
      "don't worry I will stay with you."
No, I walk with this alone.

Slowly a circle of friends formed around me after they heard the
    news
    and were able to understand it.
        Not all my old friends have made it into that circle yet
            and I am barely in that circle some days.

Inside this circle we are willing to face truth beyond denial
    find hope within hopelessness
        raw unmasked pain of a shocked and grieving heart
            knowing that some things cannot be fixed
                some things just aren't right.

There is so much I don't understand—
    so much no one else seems to understand either.
Each question to my doctor is met with paragraphs of tentative
    response scattered with "we don't really know much about this..."
I've been on the cutting edge before
    but this cutting edge is a really rough one.

Some days I wake up hating this virus that has taken me for its home
    hate it with a passion that is all-consuming.
Other days it seems OK for now since I am feeling fine these days.
    Will I ever be able to make friends with this parasite?

I actively think about killing myself
    because living with the suspense of
        something going off inside of me that I know so little about
            is just about unbearable.

This virus jams me to the brink of my own eschatological existence
    where I am confronted not only with my own end
        but also with a diminishment of my life and capacities.
            It is a wound so deep I barely can feel it.

July 29, 1988—A number of people pointed out to me that there were
two pages of obits in the *Bay Area Reporter* (a weekly gay newspaper)
this week. My, how this epidemic has grown! It is hard to keep up the
hope that AIDS doesn't mean death when the evidence mounts so
profoundly.

I also had a conversation this week with Chris which was very
disturbing. Chris and Brian came over for dinner. I had always
hesitated to invite them both over for dinner because Brian is a
professional French cook with very high standards.

Chris is a business acquaintance whom I have known for almost
ten years. We don't see each other often, but when we do, we

communicate on a deep level almost right away. He is in his late 30s I think—a solid citizen type, fun-loving and occasionally a little wild, something which I especially value in him. He works in one of the straightest jobs around. What I am trying to say is that Chris is not a crazy. He makes lots of money every year, pays taxes, and you would probably like to have him as a neighbor because he is so civic-minded about his community.

Over dinner we talked about lots of things. It is as if I have joined a club with its own set of things to talk about—T-cells, medicines, philosophy about AIDS and life, treatments, AIDS politics. At one point in the dinner, Chris says, "These people like ____ in Pennsylvania and____ in California are homophobes, and they are killing lots of people. Before I go, I am going to take a few of them with me." He is laughing loudly and I could have taken it as a joke. I didn't. I asked him what he meant exactly.

For the next hour or so he told me of his fantasy of killing some of the leaders on the political right whom he holds responsible for the failure of the government to put enough money into research to stop AIDS deaths. He said, "Their hatred is killing me and my friends, and they are going to pay. Whites didn't respond to the demands of the blacks until the Black Panthers and the Watts riots came along. It has to hurt the power establishment before they see it is in their interest to stop our dying."

"Look at all the fuss at the National Institute of Health over Legionnaire's disease—after only a few deaths! When the American Legion is dying, they do research. But the entire National Institute of Health only has 4 or 5 researchers on AIDS full-time now—after all the deaths! Thirty thousand deaths! And why? Because it is "only" gay men dying. They are glad to have us dead. Maybe I will just take a gun and kill a few of them when my T-cell count gets down around 200. What do I have to lose? I may die, but I am going to die anyway. At least I can take some of them with me."

Brian listened. He had heard this before, but Chris had never before talked about it with anyone except Brian. As we continued the discussion, it became clear that Chris had worked out quite a plan; he obviously has spent a lot of time thinking about this.

This discussion reminds me of similar ones I have had with people from liberation struggles in Africa and Central America, or from the American Indian Movement, for whom violent methods seem the only way to accomplish their ends. But here I am, confronted with my own friends, desperate and enraged—an oppressed group in my own land subjected to death and ignorance. My theory and practice in nonviolence have never been so challenged. What will it take to wake this country—this world—up? The president's commission on AIDS made lots of good recommendations; but none of them are being adopted. The president hasn't even accepted the report yet. Where is the national will to discuss, to educate, to heal, and to care?

So I present him with all the rationale I can for why things would get worse if violence started from our side. I express my bewilderment that there hasn't been more of this reactive violence. I ask Chris why he thinks it hasn't happened before. He says that when you're going to die, you are quite absorbed with getting the most out of each day, and it is hard to act. And so many people get depressed as a part of this disease—not a place from which action is easy. Both Chris and Brian complain further that the gay male community doesn't organize itself very well.

I felt very deeply his argument and point of view. I have touched within myself that place of terror and rage at the meaninglessness of this suffering. Ultimately, I say that he must do whatever he must do, and I will help him—nonviolently—in any way I can. But I shall not do anything that will encourage him to kill or physically harm anyone. Instead, I suggested some other strategies more likely to make changes, and we agreed to think more about this together in the months to come.

This is a very fine personal and strategical distinction. In no way do I condone violence. We must put all our efforts into educating people and developing empathy and intelligence about this issue. We must align ourselves with the forces of life and not death, both as we fight the virus and as we fight death-oriented forces in our society.

I have thought about this discussion a lot these past few days. This is the first time I find myself fighting for those of my own people, including myself, who are facing death. I realize that I did not decide to cast my lot with people with AIDS—in the United States, now mostly drug addicts and gay men—but life is funny that way. Now I proudly stand with them. The killing must stop. AIDS must be stopped.

The rest of the evening we spent talking about medicines, and about what Chris has learned in a year of research. When Chris and Brian first got their positive test results, they gathered a group of medical people together to figure out what to do. They had a doctor, a nurse, a researcher, and a pathologist over for dinner. The first night was really interesting, so the group decided to meet again. Chris said that the second night was a bust; there was nothing to say because they only had one night's worth of information about this disease.

July 30, 1988—In a business meeting Evelyn made some teasing comment about my intelligence, and with my new-found sensitivity it hurt my feelings. I interrupted the flow of the meeting to share this hurt and talk about what I was doing to make sure that I will be able to tell them when I am losing it. I have arranged to take a test which some researchers are giving every six months to HIV+ people to let them know that their minds are still okay, that dementia hasn't set in—or how far it has progressed if it has. Evelyn, bless her heart, said, "Fran, I think we will notice you're losing it before a test will, and we will talk to you about it." That made me think they have not yet noticed the little things I worry about as possible signs of dementia. Every time I forget anything I think quietly to myself, "Is this a sign of dementia? Oh no, I'm losing it now." Charlie always used to complain about my bad memory for short-term details. I've had this absent-mindedness for years and have done fine with it. It's the fear and self-suspicion that are the killers.

I also thought how much I love these people who I am close to, and how I rely on them for the truth—a truth that is sometimes difficult to remember myself.

July 30, 1988

International Red Cross Hospital
Peshawar, Pakistan

Dear Friends,

Two years ago, February 1987, while visiting in your area I donated blood in your hospital. I recently have found I was probably at that time carrying the AIDS virus in my blood. In May I was found to be HIV+, and I trace it back to an infection from a blood transfusion 9 years ago.

Please find whomever you gave my blood to and inform them of the risks to them and the danger they pose to others. Also, please tell them I am sincerely sorry for causing them this pain, and educate them in what is required for them so that this virus does not get going in the Afghan community. Such a valiant people have had to fight so hard, it is important that they not also have to fight this disease.

Please accept my apologies for the inconvenience this letter will cause you and all the work it will take to find the person who received my blood.

Sincerely,

Fran Peavey

Journal Entries
1988

New Friends

August 3, 1988—I cried all the way to the airport, on the way home to see my family. I had cried most of the day before too. Mimi, my doctor, has requested that I tell my family and get my durable power of attorney together—"within months, not years" she said. She doesn't want to have to break the news to my brother that I have AIDS and ask him immediately to make an intelligent decision regarding my care at that time.

For months a family reunion had been planned for early August. I was looking forward especially to meeting this J. Francis (J.F.) who had been born just before I found out about "my HIV status." Now I found myself dreading the reunion. I re-read the early entries of this journal and remembered so clearly the fight my brother and I had about AIDS. And I have to say that, with but a few exceptions, my long-time "straight" friends have not really known how to be there for me around this HIV stuff. Some have just preferred to ignore it, others continue to "go dead" when the topic comes up. People who know me don't know AIDS, and people who know AIDS haven't known me for years, so they cannot remind me of my history. Thinking about how little real sharing has been possible with most of my long-time friends did not inspire me with confidence that my family could be there with me just now as I faced this painful part of my life.

I arrived in Idaho with the idea that I was not going to talk to my family about being HIV+. But as the reunion wore on, I remembered how much I love my brother and sisters and what fine folks they really are. J.F. was a truly charming baby and I enjoyed holding him, feeding him, rocking him to sleep.

Even in this remote place, in the primitive area of Idaho, there was lots of talk about AIDS. A cousin does medical research and had lots to say. Others said they were thinking of moving back to Idaho—where there are only five cases of AIDS in the entire state—in order to protect their children. Several people asked me how it was to live in San Francisco where "there is so much AIDS going on." One cousin asked how a woman could possibly date in my city. With each question or reference to AIDS I felt embarrassed by my family's lack of education, and confused about where to begin to answer their question. Another cousin, one who digests medical information for a living, said that she had read a report that Cape Town, South Africa (a city I really love) is now 25 percent infected with HIV. Gosh that's a lot! That really saddened me.

Early in the weekend I was working along with all the other women in the kitchen. As I was cutting cabbage, I wondered how they would feel about my preparing the food they would be eating. I was especially careful with the knife.

Finally, the night before we were to go home, I decided to talk to each of my siblings. Ann was first. I am the oldest in the family and she is the next in line, three years my junior. She immediately hugged me and asked what kind of support I needed from her. She and her husband had done lots of research on AIDS because they have children. She said she would not tell her husband just now, because he is frightened and might not let me near their children—two of my favorite nephews. I really felt sad to think that I might no longer be welcome in their home and able to play with these kids whom I enjoy so much. She had a few questions and asked in a matter-of-fact way that I let her know how she could support me. I said one big way was to educate Art. She said she would.

Next was my youngest sister and her husband. It seemed best to talk to them as a unit. They are the parents of J.F. I took them behind the main cabin and we sat down. I said I wanted them to know something important that was happening in my life. As soon as I had told them, they tried to reassure me. Sue said, "Don't worry about us. I've read articles about it in women's magazines. Of course you can play with J.F. He can't get it from you—I know that." Her husband John said, "They show us lots of movies about AIDS in the Army, so I know about it." We cried a bit together, especially when we talked about how much we loved each other. They were great and said that they would help however they could.

Art, my brother, would be the tough one for me. We love each other very much but I knew this would catch him on his blind side. I walked with him over by the parking lot and told him. I saw a look cross his face that, being a Peavey, I know well. Inside that look is the thought, "Oh dear. I'm in over my head on this and likely to say something that will hurt this dear person. I'd better be very careful about what I say, try to make it brief, and hopefully I will be able to get myself squared away and talk to her again when I am less likely to say something stupid and hurt her."

I said I was naming him as my durable power of attorney along with Mike, a good friend in San Francisco. Most of all, I emphasized, I didn't want him to give Mike any shit about decisions that Mike might make in his absence. He promised.

During the entire reunion, however, I worried about the reactions of people not in my immediate family. And if I died, would they worry about my having played with their kids, cooked their food, sat on their toilet seat? Oh, I hate this suspicion and ignorance! It makes me think maybe I should just withdraw from situations where this fear could be a factor, rather than risk such a response from anyone. But where would I go?

August 10—A few days ago I found out about the details of the Dannemeyer initiative (also known as the Gann initiative or Proposition 102) in California. The initiative is named for Paul Gann who is an important political leader in California. He sponsored the tax initiative and other regressive voter initiatives. He is an old guy and is HIV+. He had a heart operation some years ago in San Francisco and drew from our blood pool. My friend Sharon, who lives up in northern California says that there are lots of older people up there with AIDS who got the virus the same way. It's a big secret. When these men and women get sick and die, they say they have cancer and not AIDS.

This ballot measure would require every HIV+ person in the state to register with the government and to disclose the names of their sexual partners. It would also force doctors and all medical people to report anyone they suspect of being HIV+ to the health department—that's the government. There is quite a stiff penalty in the initiative for failure to report sexual partners, as well as for medical personnel who refuse to report their patients.

This really frightens me. What would this allow them to do? Why does the state want my name on a list? What good would that do? Would they ultimately want to round us up and put us in camps as they did the Japanese when they believed the society was threatened in WWII? Is society going to demand that kind of protection? I have been against all such measures before. But now that I am the target, I am profoundly upset by the whole thing. It felt very different, more all-encompassing, quite terrifying actually.

Is it paranoia, or is there a hysteria building in society, one that could turn ugly? I have never felt that our society was immune to this hysteria, since I remember the persecution of the 1950s in which the communists and socialists were the target. I have read about the hysteria aimed at the anarchists in the early days of this century, and, of course, we have treated the Japanese and American Indians with this "round them up and control them" mentality in my own time. So, given our American history, I know it could happen again. But now? In this age? It seems impossible to believe.

August 1988—And Now a Word or Two about Sex. You may remember that I took this damn test three months ago because I was feeling so sexually alive and interested that I thought surely I soon would find myself in bed with one of the several people to whom I was actively attracted. I thought I could speed up that "going sexual" process by knowing that I was not carrying anything that could add an element of danger in the bedroom. More and more it is the ethic, "You want to play around? Get your test." Instead of adding security, the positive test results froze my sex drive and I found myself pulling away from people. There has been no energy for expansion—I have had to focus on getting over the shock.

This last three months I have occasionally tried to visualize how sex could be for me with the constraints of my positive status. At the lecture on women and AIDS which I attended early on, there was a section about how HIV+ women could be sexual. The lecturer said that anyone wanting to touch the vaginal areas of an infected woman should wear rubber latex gloves which are analogous to the condom. These should be used in safe sex. A 5-by-5 inch square piece of thin latex called a rubber dam was passed out. It was recommended for oral/vaginal sexual practices. If a woman or a man wanted to lick the vaginal area of an HIV+ woman, then it was recommended that this rubber dam be placed over the vaginal area first. It seemed pretty unsatisfactory to me.

In August I visited Colorado for a few days of vacation and gave a talk at a conference. I connected in a loving way at the conference with a fine woman whom I have known for over five years. We often found ourselves walking with our arms around each other. We shared deeply our concerns about the world and our love of nature. Our friendship of many years now had an added closeness, and I felt feelings of love stirring in me.

I mentioned that I needed a place to stay in Denver the one night between my meetings and my plane departure. At first she lightly offered her place and I was noncommittal. A day later she said quite directly, "I want you to come and stay with me in Denver." I met her offer evenly, "I want to come."

So it occurred that we spent the evening together. At the movie about South Africa, we nuzzled close—my arm around her shoulder, her hand on my leg. The signals of shared passion were all there. In the quiet moments I wondered how I could possibly enter the sexual land with her. I had not brought latex gloves. I couldn't see myself using a rubber dam, and I was conflicted by fear, desire, and lack of planning. In some ways this evening reminded me of the night I lost my virginity. There was all that unknowing and awkwardness. Fortunately, she seemed relatively assured and at ease.

I had told her of my HIV+ status a few days earlier, and that had not seemed to inhibit her getting close to me. In fact, I worried that maybe it was a factor propelling her toward me. Could it be that she felt sorry for me? I decided to put suspicions aside as I had no evidence for them.

As bedtime approached, we both grew very quiet, each working out in her own mind what we wanted to do and questioning how it could be done. The question of sex hung "pregnant" in the air. I undressed in my bedroom, and she in hers. Wearing my bathrobe, I ventured into her bedroom to say "good night." I found her dressed in her bathrobe sitting quietly on a bench, her hands folded. I put my arm around her shoulder. I wanted very much to hold her but was unsure if anything beyond that would be possible for me without me freaking out. I might as well admit that. I was deeply afraid of sex at that moment, or even of bringing up those feelings, with so much confusion and fear surrounding sex in my mind.

As we fell into each other's arms I tried to ascertain where she was on the issue of kissing and her level of knowledge about the virus and sexual behaviors. She mentioned that kissing was out because she had just had her teeth cleaned that day. Her gums would be sore and any virus in my saliva could take that opportunity to get into her blood system. I was impressed that she knew about the effect of teeth-cleaning on her susceptibility for infection. (When getting ready for bed I had deliberately not brushed my teeth or flossed because of the possibility of disturbing my gums and bringing blood with its virus into my mouth.)

Somewhere she had gotten the idea that it was dangerous for either of us to touch each other in the vaginal area. I explained in a surprisingly (to me at least) reasoned and calm way that it was not dangerous to her for me to touch her (providing my hands were not bleeding, of course); but the danger lay in her touching my vaginal area without a latex glove on her hand.

It was fine loving that night. We found safe ways of opening further and further to each other. Each opening had a wholeness to it that was just plain fun. Somehow in spite of our mutual reservations we proceeded through several delightful orgasms. At one point, in the thick of emotion, she approached my vaginal area with her hand, and I stopped her. Acknowledging how deeply I wished to have her touch that center, I had to say that it would not be safe for her. Immediately I was filled with a sense of relief that I would be able to take care of her even in the face of my desire.

There were several moments in the night where I was painfully aware of the costs of being HIV+. I would have loved to kiss her deeply for a long time—but that was not a good idea, especially with her gums being sore. I would have loved to have her touch me in the deepest way, but that was not possible for now until we got a glove. And of course, there were places I could not lick, kiss, and enjoy—the same places she could not lick, kiss, and enjoy as women have done for centuries together.

All of this denial of pleasure occurred inside a framework of my suspicion that it might not really be necessary at all. There have only been two instances of woman-to-woman infection at this point in history, and one of those was doubtful. But how does one evaluate this evidence and make responsible choices? If I ignore the medical advice available at this time and go ahead and do what I want to do and thereby infect someone, what kind of crime is that? Would she ever forgive me? Would I if I were in her shoes? Probably not. If I had someone to blame all this suffering on, I would be pretty pissed. Would I ever forgive myself if through my casualness, she were to contract such a dangerous disease?

One particular experience may serve to illuminate many aspects of living with HIV. She is lying on my breast, we are quietly talking. With her finger she lightly strokes a place high on my breast where I have two small reddish blue spots. I have been secretly worrying if those are pozies for some time, but I have been embarrassed to bring up the subject with my doctor. I don't want to be one of those patients who runs to the doctor with every little blemish. And besides, I am not sure I want to know if the information is bad. It would be a great relief if it was simply a—well, something else. But I don't feel ready for that risk.

So this is what runs through my mind as she strokes this area. "Does she notice the spot? Of course she does, the lights are on and she is not blind. Does she think it is a pozie? Is it a pozie? I don't know. I can't remember when it came. It hasn't been long—but then again, maybe it's been a year or so. Why can't I remember these things?" Then I get on the downward spiral of wondering about my mind. "Is it going now—right now as I am lying here, is it going?"

Because the mind is a closed system, the only way to get off that spiral is either to exert great mental discipline or talk about it. I, more often than not, lack the mental discipline as well as the courage to share what is really going on for me at the moment. So I re-enter the present time with a five-to-ten minute blip in my being fully present, wondering what I missed, hoping no one noticed my absence.

Early in the morning, I had to catch a plane. As she drove me to the airport we quietly held hands. I noticed a sore on her hand and a mini-terror gripped me. What if I had allowed her to continue her approach to my vagina and a virus had entered her system through that little hole? I felt so sad at the possibility, angry that she had not believed that she had to protect herself, and relieved that I had been able to protect both of us.

Now as I write this several days later, I am filled with grief for the very real sexual practices I have enjoyed in my past and which now are lost. A friend just called to ask if I would like to go see some sex videos tomorrow. A wave of sadness and jealousy swept over me. No, I don't want to see how other women can make love when I can't. I don't want to be reminded of what I have lost. It is too hard. I want to build an image bank of what I *can* be—what I *can* do—not what is denied to me. I have to put out the energy to keep from being too discouraged and depressed.

Please bear with me through this next part because in all good conscience I have to put this information in here. I thought I knew all the facts but when the wave hit me in May, I realized I was not entirely clear about some key facts about how you get AIDS. I have been collecting reliable information to my questions. Please read it. We'll get back to the journal in a few pages.

Because I wouldn't want to be the route for this virus to travel to anyone else, I have spent quite a bit of energy researching how these little buggers get passed around. I have confidence in this research. What's more, I have talked to enough people about their own information—and rampant misinformation—to know there is a crying need for more education and confidence-building with respect to this research. This may be the most vital information you can learn these days if you are at all sexually active, or your partner is, or your children are, or if you have ever wondered about the safety of eating in restaurants, sitting on toilets, touching or kissing people.

Let's start with a basic understanding of the virus itself. If you keep clearly in mind what is known about its properties, you will have a framework for thinking about the ways it can and cannot be spread.

As I've said before, AIDS is not easy to get. The virus has to be transmitted directly into the blood stream. It can get there by three paths: blood to blood, semen to blood, or vaginal juices to blood. That's It!

The virus can't enter the blood from the digestive tract, or from the lungs; therefore you can't get AIDS from food or from breathing in San Francisco. You also can't get it from hugs, bicycle seats, hot tubs, toilet seats, sharing a glass, eating food prepared by a person with AIDS, sitting next to an HIV+ person on the bus, being breathed or sneezed upon, or mosquito bites. This represents a remarkable consensus of scientific studies on all continents. The transmission routes by which AIDS travels are unforgiving, but we don't need to fantasize about new, esoteric ones besides.

A small number of health care workers have been infected by this virus, and they have all had some blood-to-blood contact such as accidentally sticking themselves with a syringe that has HIV+ blood in it.

I have heard of people who have stopped going to restaurants out of fear that HIV+ food handlers might spread AIDS. This really can't happen. Even if an infected food handler were to bleed directly on your food and be so perverse or blind as to serve it anyway, the virus would be killed by any of the following: the heat of cooking, the acidity of the food, the time elapsed between the bleeding and the serving, and the action of your digestive juices.

One of the most agonizing questions, of course, is whether HIV+ children can infect their peers while playing and roughhousing. Researchers have applied their most rigorous analysis to this data, and here's what they say: not a single case has been found of siblings or other family members (not sexual partners) getting the virus this way. It has not happened.

When we say that the AIDS virus is transmitted by blood contact, it does not mean you must be bleeding to be infected. Healthy skin will protect your blood stream from the virus. But if you have a sore, a pimple, or open sore gums, or chapped hands that are not yet fully healed, then direct contact with contaminated blood or semen or vaginal juices on those areas can let the virus into your blood.

The AIDS virus is extremely fragile outside the body. It needs a warm, moist human body to live in. It dies within minutes after leaving that protected environment.

If AIDS is so hard to get, why are so many people getting it? Because they don't take the risk seriously, or because they encountered the virus before they encountered the information which is the greatest protection against it. Here are the main ways people get AIDS:

- unsafe sex with an HIV+ person (i.e. sex that does not protect against any kind of exchange of blood-semen-vaginal juices);
- sharing needles with people who have the virus;
- infected blood products (a major problem before March of 1985, when blood banks began carefully testing their supplies and rejecting any blood that shows positive or questionable test results);
- exposure of a baby before birth to an HIV+ mother.

To stop this virus, then, men and women need to be tested as they are entering into sexual relations.

Please be careful with your sex life. Most of all, those of us on this HIV path do not want to share it with you. We are human beings, though, so we may not always be on our guard. Protect yourself. Don't expect others to protect you. Life—yours and all life—is worth a little bit of latex and care.

Much has been written about the use of a condom for anyone—a woman or a man—loving a man. It is necessary now, in order to control this virus, to use these latex forms of protection until the status of your lover is known and a basis of trust is established so you can be confident that he is not out getting the virus from someone else.

Because so few women have been visible in the AIDS picture until recently, there has not been much attention given to what precautions are necessary for a man or woman loving a HIV+ woman—or anyone whose HIV status you aren't sure of. Safe sex includes using a rubber glove when stroking a woman's vaginal area. All lovers of women need to use a rubber dam when enjoying oral sex. Although the concentration of HIV in normal day-to-day vaginal moisture isn't high enough to transmit the virus, the concentration becomes dangerously high before and after a woman's period, and while she is lubricating and experiencing orgasm.

What about kissing? Well, the AIDS virus is rarely found in saliva at all, and it almost certainly does not have a high enough concentration of the virus to transmit AIDS to another person. Experts are still being careful about saying kissing is 100 percent safe. But things like pecks on the mouth, lip nibbling, and sucking are thought to be safe. Deep penetrating kisses — the kind that are the greatest fun — are the most questionable, especially if a lot of saliva is exchanged.

Now, if you're reading this and you're shooting up drugs, I hope you will find a way to stop. But if you're not ready to do that yet, before using someone else's needle, put bleach (Clorox or some other brand) into the needle and shoot it out. Then wash out the bleach from the needle with clean water. *Do this twice.* It's important to do this, because you want to live long enough to enjoy life, and not having the virus inside you gives you the best chance of living that long.

That's it. That's all the ways the HIV fire is spreading through our species. So, give yourself a break. Stop worrying about the esoteric ways of getting AIDS. Just use safe sex, don't share needles, and stay out of the way of blood.

The job of educating people about how AIDS is spread has been remarkably effective. In San Francisco the rate of new infections in the gay community is 1 percent. But the real story of successful education came from my nephew, who is eight years old. He was watching a televised report of Gary Hart's troubles during the 1988 campaign. He went to his mother to ask why Hart was in such trouble. "Well," his mother said, "he's married and he spent the night with another woman." My nephew replied without missing a beat, "What's the matter? Didn't he use a condom?"

Back to the Journal

August 26—The Pain Ripples out Further. I was talking about sex with a previous partner, Karla. She mentioned to me that the woman she was sleeping with these days had freaked out when Karla had said she'd been involved with someone who later tested positive. Although Karla had tested negative for the virus and was sure that she couldn't pass it on, the woman freaked out about it and assumed she would probably get AIDS. She withdrew sexually from Karla and went through a major trauma over the whole thing.

How confident can we be about these tests? Is Karla really negative, or is the virus lying latent, waiting to go off inside her? How long before they can really be sure?

And how do I know for sure that I am positive? What if they made a mistake or something? Sometimes I go through what I call the "loop of infinite uncertainty." Maybe I should get another set of tests. But then if the results were positive I would just be bummed out all over again. I don't think I could go through that again. And if the results were negative, which results would I believe: the four that were positive or the four that were negative? How many tests would I have to take before I could believe one or the other?

I could spend my whole life trying to get some more certainty about this. What would give certainty? And how would that impact my life? Nothing can erase this blot on my blood, it seems. But I do keep thinking about getting another set of tests—or ten.

A Few Days Later—Oh, what heavy days! There seem to be a number of factors creating this hysterical weight I feel: (1) I allowed someone to get close enough to see some of the dysfunctional parts of my body and the correlating dysfunctional parts of my denial system; (2) I completed a whole battery of neurological tests which convinced me that there is something not so together about my legs; (3) a poll I read about reported that over 70 percent of the voters in California say they will vote for the Paul Gann Public Health Act, also known as the Dannemeyer initiative; (4) I feel so alone in my thinking and confusion; (5) I do not feel like myself.

I am uncharacteristically ambivalent, so crumpled that I do not recognize myself. How will I take care of myself and help myself think in the face of such confusion? I am so confused lately that even to start making decisions reminds me of so many other decisions I must make that it seems overwhelming.

I don't even recognize myself these days. This is not like me. I am usually quite decisive. But now I cannot decide on anything. When shall I go to South Africa? Where shall I live for the next period of my life? God, I hate this part! I NEVER THOUGHT THIS WOULD BE HAPPENING TO ME, AND I DON'T LIKE IT!

With all of this rolling around inside me, plus still grieving somewhat over the loss of possibilities in my sexual menu, I spent a few sleepless nights. Finally, on Thursday I concluded that I was in trouble with myself and was heading into dangerous emotional waters. It seemed I had the choice of either going crazy or making a plan. Facing this crisis, I made a plan: (1) I would see one of my doctors that day, no matter how hard it would be to get an appointment. (2) I would figure out a way to let more of my social context into my real situation. A possibility is my birthday party which is coming up. I could talk to friends there and let them know that I am not doing as well as they might think from seeing my functioning self. (3) I should have a vacation away from all this stuff.

With new determination and a real sense of purpose I went in to finish up the neurological tests I had been unable to complete the day before. The tests were usually given in an eight-hour battery, and I am not sure why it took me twelve hours to do the whole protocol. I had also lost some of the key papers I had spent hours filling out for the test. I had to do them over before my 7:30 a.m. meeting on Friday to finish up the tests. I have always joked that I have a paper allergy because I lose so many papers. With this newfound anxiety over my mental state, losing anything becomes a threat to my self-confidence.

On Thursday I had worked hard at the tests, but I told the doctor at the beginning of the appointment that it was a low day for me. Finally she stopped the tests and kindly asked me if I could tell her a little about what was bothering me. It all came pouring out. I felt very shaky and just sobbed when I told her of my worries and how tired I was.

While I was in the testing office I saw a phone list of people on the AIDS neurological testing staff. There must have been over twenty names on that list. I thought of all the offices I had visited in the last four months, and how many workers must be employed in the testing, research, and care of AIDS/HIV+ people in this city. It is truly a growth industry! AIDS must be one of the biggest employers in San Francisco at this time.

On Friday I called my doctor, Mimi, at SF General Hospital. With determination carefully placed in my voice, I said as clearly as I could, "I need to see you today." I knew how impossible that was, given her schedule, but I also knew how impossible it was for me to go on. She met me where I was. "Come at 1:10," she said. "We may be interrupted by medical students needing advice, but I will see you."

I quickly made a list of my worries and called Karen to see if she could go with me. She reports that I screamed hysterically for an hour and a half about my concerns. It didn't seem that long to me, but I was definitely beyond control.

Soon after I arrived, Mimi came to the waiting room to get me. When I sat down in her office I hardly knew where to begin. She did some more tests and said that it was true that I had mild peripheral neuropathy, and that I would need a brace on my leg to keep from stumbling. This could be related to the virus or perhaps not. She said it was about 60 percent likely that it was HIV-related neuropathy. Whatever the reason, the nerves that tell my foot to come up as I walk aren't working, and I have what they call "foot drop." When I asked if I could exercise and get it back, she just looked at me quizzically. But the most important thing she said—and she said it right away and in several different ways so I really could hear it—was, "Just because the virus has attacked your peripheral nervous system does not mean that it has or will attack your central nervous system." She also said the neuropathy could be caused by other factors such as diabetes. We checked my blood sugar and it was well within the normal range.

I showed her the marks on my breast. She said they didn't look like pozies to her, but that if they didn't go away in a few weeks we would biopsy them. The renewed pain in my gut, as well as a few other minor complaints, we would have to look at later.

I hate being obsessed with these physical worries. I have noticed this is almost characteristic of HIV+ people—every little mark, every pain is a source of upset and preoccupation. This is natural, I guess. I realize that I need to know when to begin to fight with drugs— when I have gone from the latency stage to the stage when the virus is active. The earlier the treatment starts, the better the results. And so one is always nervous and on guard.

Mimi was firm and short concerning my doubts about giving up certain sexual practices, even though only two cases of woman-to-woman transmission have been reported. Men have been infected from women and we know the virus is found in vaginal fluids. It is just that the virus has not gotten a hold in the lesbian community, so it has not spread there. I must practice safe sex.

But the real victory was talking to her about the Gann initiative. I asked her what she was going to do. "I haven't been tracking that initiative much. I don't think it will pass, do you?" I told her about last week's California Field poll, in which over 70 percent of the voters said that they would vote for it. She looked at me soberly and asked, "Are you asking me if I will report you?" "Yes," I replied, feeling very scared of her answer and the risk of the moment. It felt like a sacred moment in our relationship, a moment where I needed her to make a vow that she hadn't really thought through.

She looked at me squarely. "I promise you I will not report you to anyone." Those were her exact words. I even remember how they sounded, so important they were to me.

August 28, Sunday—Traditionally, around my birthday I have a party for my friends and do what I call a "General Accounting." I cook a whole salmon, others bring potluck, and we feast on a great dinner. Then I introduce each person to the group, sharing what I treasure about our relationship. Next I give a little speech. I talk about the past year, the victories and difficulties, and what I look forward to in the upcoming year. I describe what kind of help I anticipate I will need to do the things I will be doing in the coming year. Since I do not have a boss as such, living mainly as a social change artist doing work that "calls me," I need to be accountable to someone for my vision and my standard of excellence in my work. Each year it is also helpful for me to articulate my social dream, and what facet of that dream I am working with just now to bring that dream into reality. Different years have been focused on residential hotels for poor people, work with self-determination for alcoholics and street people, planning and executing major campaigns against nuclear weapons and power plants. And there is always my continuing work to clean the Ganges River in India every winter. My social dreams center around justice, environmental harmony, and respect for diversity.

Often in the middle of the year, in those moments when I waver in my direction, I think of the people who stand with me in support of my work. Sometimes I'm in war zones and think I should leave rather than do my job there. Or sometimes the variety of political groups and infighting is just too complex and frustrating and I think of leaving that struggle for something less ambiguous. How will I explain this to my friends at my next general accounting? I don't want to let them down. So I think of this activity as a sort of reporting to the employers who hold me accountable for my work in the world. It is a great social invention, and I always appreciate people's willingness to go along with it. The invitees seem to have a good time with each other too. I think it reminds them of their social dreams which so easily get lost in our busy lives.

On Thursday night, in the midst of my personal black hole, I concluded that one thing had to change: I had to break the system of secrecy and isolation that I had built around myself and my HIV battles. This system had come to seem dangerous to me. I was protecting my long-term friends from what was really happening to me, relying on an entirely too shallow support base of only a few people who knew about AIDS. I had reflected many times on my observation that "the people who know me don't know AIDS, and the people who know AIDS don't know me and can't remind me of who I am historically." Rather than educating my long-time friends about the HIV-positive issues I was struggling with, I huddled with newer friends who knew about AIDS and had already worked through much of their fear.

In response to my invitation I received this note in my computer mail box from a dear friend and wise person, Bob:

> Alia [his wife] won't get back from Marin with the car till about 8pm tonight. So coming then doesn't make sense... Meanwhile, Evelyn tells me some of your woes. As for leg braces, I would try some leg strengthening exercises with a Nautilus-type machine first. I do it a few times a week at the UC-Berkeley gym, but these machines are now everywhere and there is a free, simple alternative with huge rubber straps that go from the ankle to a heavy table leg that you pull against. The thing to do about physical deterioration is to fight it. Fighting is fun. I have been at it for several years and as I get slower it gets to be more fun, surprisingly. I shall try for a 51-year personal record on Tuesday. You could try for a 45-year Fran record; and then a 46, etc. I know you like a good battle. Same for the stupid Gann initiative. Battle it—use yourself up so when you go you're spent fully—that is the only satisfaction I can find. I remember a famous old prof of English at Princeton who, standing in his garden one day, pointed to the humus pile and said, 'That is all I am, humus.' On the one hand he meant that he was shit; on the other he meant that he was fertile soil for other living things to grow in after he was gone. One could do worse than be a pile of humus! HAPPY BIRTHDAY. LOVE BOB.

By Sunday I had my head enough out of the muck to begin to get a clearer picture of what I wanted to do. The people I had invited were all those whom I trusted enough by that point to have told about my HIV+ status, or as I have come to refer to it, "my situation."

When folks gathered in the upstairs room for the General Accounting, I began by saying that this would not be a regular accounting, because I found it impossible to remember much about the pre-HIV+ year just now. I talked briefly about how my work went in India this year, how deeply satisfying my relationships with the India group were, and how the fact that the river was getting perceptibly cleaner in our lifetime seemed a miracle. So rarely does one see much material results for social change work. I also mentioned how much it had meant to me that Charlie and I had peacefully laid to rest our eight-year performing career together.

Then—as I remember it—I took a big breath and started to talk about how hard the HIV+ life has been for me. I told this group how confused I was, how difficult decisions were for me now, how I didn't even recognize myself these days. I talked about the news of being potentially "a few smt's," and about how hard it was for me to let them see my own fear and alienation from them. I said clearly that I was going to need their help, without really knowing at this point what that means. For now, at least, I needed not to have to be okay for them, and I needed help in planning and thinking through things that were complex and distressing for me. Should I move to less expensive housing with fewer steps and a level garden? Should I continue to work in third world countries where I would be more likely to be exposed to infections which would challenge my immune system? So many questions.

In that room sat some people worried about their own status, others facing their own tests in the near future, and others who already knew they were HIV+ but were not able to be open about it. This epidemic touches everyone whether or not they realize it.

Terry spoke of her gratitude to me for being open about my condition and feelings. She said that more than ten of her friends had died in the last several years, and none of them have even told her what they were going through or that they had AIDS. She had felt cut off from loving them in the way she would have liked to, and she felt they didn't trust her.

Next I turned to the Gann initiative and shared how this looked to me. If HIV+ people are driven underground, if medical care becomes a way for them to be turned in to the government, then most people will not get tested and the epidemic will spread. And as it spreads, will the society ultimately feel it needs to control us in some way? And if so, what will that way be? And isn't registration the first step towards any of those subsequent steps? Carlene spoke about it too, comparing our situation to Nazi Germany. Everyone got a copy of a leaflet about the initiative as they left the party.

At various times in the evening, laughter filled the room. The mood was not at all grim. Albert said he had been to jollier parties—everyone laughed. Several people offered to facilitate a group for people who wanted to learn more about AIDS and explore their own feelings. I knew people were going to be better able to "step into the circle" with me from now on, and I felt warmed and heartened by their support. I felt I had broken at least a piece of the system of denial and pretense that had had me in its grip.

August 29. The Next Day—The sun is out now, and except for occasionally wishing that one could have cats in the bags as well as out, I am feeling fine about the sharing I did last night and the love and support I felt afterwards. I worried that I have been too self-absorbed and preoccupied with my own condition, and that it was occupying too much of my perceptual field. I vowed to work more this week on thinking of ways I can tune in more to the needs of others and offer support for their battles. I also spent at least two hours designing a little exercise machine to start working on my legs to get them stronger. I think it can be done.

I am up for any battle I can understand.

September 1, 1988—Andora's ex-husband died of AIDS last week, Mike tells me. He says that there are now people dying who are friends. Since the funerals would involve the same group of people, they are bunching up the memorial services and having one service for two or three friends at the same time.

This reminds me of a story Jim, the minister at our church, told recently. He was presiding at a funeral of an activist who had died of AIDS. The dead man had requested in his funeral instructions that china plates be broken at his funeral. He was angry about death. He knew others at the funeral would be angry about all the dying. Jim said that initially he was intimidated by such an angry act, and hesitatingly flung the first plate into the fireplace. He was surprised at how releasing it felt. Looking at the faces of the others as they dashed the plates, he could feel the pent up anger in this community about so many funerals—so many friends gone.

Michael Callen, a PWA in an album called *Purple Heart* has some appropriate lyrics:

I know what it's like to have a graveyard as a friend
    'cause that's where they are, boy—all of them.
Don't seem likely I'll get friends like them again.
But it's time I've moved on
We are living—we are living in war time
We are living—it's just our grieving in war time.
More die every day.
This is war.
    This is war.

Journal Entries

1988

September 3—Today I awoke from my nap with two clear thoughts. One was that if they ask all the HIV+ people to register and tell their previous partners, everyone who is negative should go en masse to the registration office and register. I have heard the story of King Christian of Denmark in World War II. The German army invaded and decreed that all Jews were to wear a yellow star of David. In the morning, so the story goes, the king came out on his horse for a ride through town wearing a yellow star; by afternoon the citizenry had followed suit. Now it was impossible to tell the Jews from everyone else, so the order lost its punch.

If hundreds or even thousands of people went to register, it would make the Gann initiative impossible to enforce. Maybe they should name Governor Deukmajian or Ronald Reagan as their sexual partners or people they had been fucked by. Then the registration would be meaningless as well as impossible. The main problem with this is that the society's need to be protected would still not be acknowledged. The hysteria would only build.

I don't know why people think that something should occur besides each person protecting her- or himself with safe sex. People always like to think that the resolution of problems lies beyond themselves, but in this instance it is very clear—the only meaningful protection is changing one's own behavior.

My other thought was that AIDS is not really *caused* by sex and that we have to labor to teach people that. The AIDS virus is *spread* by sexual contact (among other ways) but it is *caused* by some deadly mutation of a virus. Now the real question is why has this virus mutated like this? Is it a natural mutation in the long line of evolution, or does it arise out of an increasingly destroyed radioactive environment which encourages mutations? I wonder if we have built a world we cannot live in. Focusing on sex is misplaced fear. Why are people so upset about AIDS? Maybe it is in part because we fear that AIDS is a sign—no longer avoidable—that we cannot live the lifestyle to which we have become addicted. We need food that is not injected with hormones and pesticides. We need the forests, we need ozone in the stratosphere, we need clean water, and on and on it goes. Deep inside of each being is the knowledge that we cannot live without these things. Yet we are destroying them.

I just don't know why this new disease is with us now. Could it be that the levels of radiation in our environment cause mutations in things like bacteria and viruses? Or is our immunity being destroyed by these designer drugs we put into our bodies for every infection we get as we grow up? And what about the antibiotics and pesticides we ingest in our foods? What effect do they have? Some people suggest that this is not a new disease, but is an old bug now finding the new situation of people with weak immune systems. I don't know, but there is lots of speculation on the streets and in the press about the origins of this virus. Some conspiracy theorists think the CIA invented this disease and planted it in the gay community and in Africa. Others suggest it was developed in Jonestown.

But most of us really don't know, and it is disquieting to live and die within such a mystery.

September 4—I went to Mike and Catherine's house for dinner tonight. Three others were also invited. Two of the three were people very involved in sex education work in the early seventies. I expected that it would be a fine time, reminiscing and telling funny stories about the good old days. Three of the people in the room knew my status and three did not. And today I was not interested in talking about it.

As this evening wore on, one thing became very obvious: it is impossible to escape AIDS talk in this epidemic. Mike and Catherine knew I was not wanting to talk about AIDS. Yet the topic came up three times in normal conversation, never originated by any of the three of us. When we did not contribute to the discussion of an AIDS-related topic, after a few minutes the conversation would switch to another subject. But AIDS kept coming back into the conversation, three times in all.

I have noticed this so many times that I think it is worth noting here. Individuals who are deeply disturbed by a wound in the social fabric of which they are a part tend to talk obsessively about this collective wound, as if they could discharge the emotion around the subject and thereby figure it out. No wonder I feel surrounded by AIDS. It's in the newspapers and on TV. I see notices on telephone poles about AIDS groups and therapies. It's in every conversation. How can I escape?

September 11, 1988—A wonderful piece of sex research was done for me by two dear friends yesterday. They played around with a rubber dam and latex glove, researching what safe sex with an HIV+ woman would be like. They reported it was every bit as satisfying for the partner being licked, but the licker was not as sensually satisfied. Even though the dam was vanilla-flavored, the taste was not sensuous and the fun was reduced. They said just make sure there is a liquid base under the dam so suction can be achieved.

Their review of latex gloves was that the experience was fine for the touchee, but for the toucher the sensation was definitely cut down. This is similar to what men report about a condom. Overall, it was a glowing and encouraging report. And now that more women are getting this virus, this information will be of use to men and women loving HIV+ women.

Also at church, some guys from my new HIV+ support group (the women's support group ended) came up and were teasing—accusing me of losing their phone numbers since I had not called them for support. We were laughing, hugging, and carrying on like old friends.

Then, very quietly and without the others noticing it, one of them turned to me and said, "You know, they are saying we should get guns and protect ourselves. What do you think?" Time stopped. We sat down and talked deeply about his despair, about all his friends who had died, and about how tired and fed up with it all he was. A friend of his joined us and the three of us talked about the "violent solution."

You see, no one really thinks that getting our names registered on a list will be the end of it, if the Gann initiative passes. These lists will be a way to watch us, possibly to place us in hospitals or somewhere else where we can't infect the rest of the population. And to turn our doctors (who know so little about how to help us anyway) against us is really adding insult to injury. Other people could report anyone they even suspected of being HIV+, and then we are all—even you— surrounded in a climate of suspicion and hostility.

Well, it is just real difficult to feel good about that. It feels wrong— terribly wrong. And it seems to me that it will only drive many of us underground, with more alienation from the society and with less likelihood that we will act in a responsible fashion with our "bodily fluids." The disease will spread faster and farther.

On the way to a brunch, I picked up a *Sentinel* and read this article, which was featured prominently:

Searching for Hope in the Midst of Crisis: Standing on the Titanic
By Krandall Kraus

Like so many people these days, I am feeling nearly at the end of my emotional rope. This weekend, as I sat with my partner (who is barely able to get out of bed most days) talking about the death of his closest friend Clark, I realized I have lost count of the number of friends and acquaintances who have succumbed to AIDS and to this nation's indifference.

In the past few days I have had another realization just as startling and frightening: My surviving friends are less and less able to support and comfort one another. They try. They make themselves available and go through all the motions, but more and more often there is less and less to give as they struggle to hold their own lives together. Not only am I as an individual fading in my ability to cope; we, as a community, are approaching, if not the end of our collective emotional, financial, and political lifeline, certainly the last frayed strings.

It feels to me lately that we are all standing on the deck of a modern-day Titanic. A small number (mostly women and children, ironically) have managed to secure a place in a lifeboat, although not all of them shall survive, either. Some at the unlucky end of the ship have already drowned. The rest of us are either watching the water slowly rise around our necks or are waiting at the high end of the deck, wondering how long it will take for the sea to reach us. As the ship slowly submerges, we are becoming increasingly aware that there is little if anything we can do for ourselves, little if anything we can do for one another. And our mood is changing. After all, we can only smile and sing anthems for so long....

Over 30,000 people have died slow, painful deaths. Over 30,000 more are dying as I write this. Are we really such a cold, uncaring people that we will not reach out—if not to help, at least to comfort?...

Already groups of militant PWAs are forming and demonstrating. What kind of a society produces such a phenomenon? Has there ever been another time in history when the terminally ill had to become militant in order to get help? If such laws as Proposition 102 (the Gann initiative) are passed, will there be any recourse for us but to resort to violence when they try to blacklist us and eventually "round us up"? Don't they realize the volatility of our situation? There are over 30,000 people diagnosed with AIDS and tens of thousands more with ARC who have nothing to lose by arming themselves and doing battle with those who would deny them their rights and hasten their deaths. It is an ugly alternative, yet it is an alternative which I will not run from if all else fails.

Now the violence I have been sniffing in the air has found its way into print.

It's a long walk home—one I rarely do. But today was one of those days I felt like walking. As I reached the top of Castro Street, I looked back at the Castro district and at my city. This city has been my home for twenty-seven years. How I love San Francisco! It has been very good to me. But this love is also tinged with bitterness—it has become the source for me of this new pain.

September 11, 1988—Visiting a friend who knows I am HIV+, we drink a cup of tea. When we prepare to leave, he comes in and shyly says, "I'm embarrassed to ask, but do you do anything special with your dishes?" I felt a bit stigmatized and embarrassed myself. "No," I reply. "The virus doesn't live long outside my body. Just wash the cup with soap and water." We go on without missing a beat in our conversation.

Tuesday, September 13—The HIV+ women's support group I had attended for two months ended; the rules set by the city, which sponsors the group, prohibit anyone staying in the group longer than two months. So in July I checked out another group which meets at church, which is (or was until I joined) composed of all men. So far I have attended two meetings of this all-men-plus-me HIV+ support group.

Last night's HIV+ support group was interesting. We met at the pastor's home. He is a gay man who freely admits that he has not been tested. But he sits with us one night a month and mostly listens. It feels a little strange being the only woman, but I am getting less shy—a difference which was noticeable to me and to them.

These guys really extend themselves to make me feel welcome. Sometimes I think I may know a little how blacks feel coming into white groups. These men are *very* nice to me, and I do appreciate how they tease me and joke. We opened the group by sharing our first names (we are an anonymous group in principle at least), and one victory we'd had in the last month. Some people had been on vacations. Several had recently come out to their parents, either as being gay or HIV+.

A number of people had gotten "their numbers" this month. (This means, in AIDS-ese, their T-cell counts.) The people who shared on this subject had higher numbers this counting time than last time. Murmurs of "congratulations," "way to go" could be heard after each report. Others said how much they dreaded getting their T-cell tests done.

I talked about some of my recent experiences described in these journals. There was lots of good-natured laughter about my sexual experience. One man said, "Good for you! Sex keeps your numbers up. Safe sex of course!" So many of the men have talked about how fraught with anxiety and fear dating is, and how difficult sex is for them with the changes which are required by our new status. Many of them forego sex altogether.

Next there was time for each of the twelve of us to say what was on our minds this month. Several people spoke of fighting deep loneliness, and about how hard it was to face these times alone. Others mentioned fear of discovery of their status on the job, and their struggle to find a good doctor who both understood AIDS and would take on new patients.

One man admitted that he feels "stained or tainted." He said it is a struggle to feel good about himself on a minute-to-minute basis while feeling stained. Judging by the nods in the room and murmurs of agreement, I would guess that many of us identified with this feeling. It seems odd how much shame there is surrounding this illness. But I feel that stain inside me too. I think it's why that crumpled feeling has replaced my general state of okay-ness these last few months. And I hate it. That a person like me—or like them—should feel shame about this shows that something is wrong. They tell us how we catch the virus, but they do not mention how shame, which is equally damaging, arises. In my entire life I have not been prone to such feelings.

Many people discussed their struggle to control stress and their frequent attacks of anxiety. This discussion was overlaid with lots of talk about vitamins, various drugs and treatments and where to get them, and meditation/prayer campaigns. After each person had a chance to speak, we went around and each shared a goal we had for ourselves this next month. Mine was to find a way to reduce stress and improve my concentration.

Occasionally when people spoke very much from the heart, I would feel tears well up in my eyes. We are up against such odds, and it is so hard sometimes. And yet these really beautiful spirits are finding their way through it all. And some of them freely say these times are some of the best they have had in their whole lives. Some have cleaned up their drinking and drug habits, and some are experiencing a level of intimacy previously unknown to them. I am again reminded of the way men talk about war—living at their very edge, relying on their buddies for life itself.

But especially during the closing prayer, I feel my eyes go damp when Jim says, "God knows you by name." Tears freely flow down my face as it occurs to me that so many of us feel forced to have these secret identities and to live secret lives.

September 14, 1988—I went to the doctor today. Mimi did more tests on my feet. This visit was calmer than the last one. We talked about my getting shots as I prepare to travel soon for my work. I must be careful because my immune system may not be able to handle living viruses such as those in yellow fever shots. Mimi also reminded me that there is a growing list of countries which won't let you in if you are HIV+. I know this is true of India regarding long-term visas, but so far not for tourist visas. My world is shrinking. This saddens me.

Mimi did more testing of my feet and legs. She said that neuropathy could be caused by many things, including MS or diabetes. But she gave odds of 60 percent that it was HIV-related neuropathy. I still don't know how this virus can affect the nerves and make them hurt, as well as inhibiting the messages telling my foot to move. But evidently, this is common. In any event, I should be careful about it spreading, because it could be serious if it begins to affect my lungs.

It is deeply disappointing to me that I can have a great T-cell count and still have neuropathy. The T-cell count relates to the immune system, while neuropathy involves the nervous system.

Then we discussed whether or not to biopsy these spots. Of course they were still there. Mimi said she did not think they looked like Kaposi's spots to her. I asked her, "If they were your spots would you have them biopsied?" She diplomatically replied, "I wouldn't, but if I were HIV+ I don't know what I would do. I would want to know for sure, I think." I asked what could be done if they were pozies. She said that there was little they could do to treat the spots or me, but that they could then diagnose me.

This "diagnose" business is bad. It means that one has moved from 0 smt to ARC or AIDS. I asked cynically, "Why would that be to my advantage?" "Oh," she responded, "You could get on welfare and be eligible for some programs." I said I don't need to be labeled for the government or for anyone else, thank you.

Somehow I have to find out about this new medicine which I hear is being tested somewhere in the city. I hear it blocks the virus from entering the nerve cells. It is in the experimentation phase, and Mimi doesn't know about it yet. In the hospital there is an office where you can find out all about the latest treatments and experiments if you let them study you or your blood. But I have limited time for such appointments. I have my life and my work and I really do not want to have this virus take over my entire life. And I feel fine these days.

From what I hear, if you do participate in one of these experimental programs, only half of the people in the study get the medicine. The other half gets a placebo (doctor language for "nothing"). So one half gets something which may or may not help, and the other half of the people (these are human beings who someone probably loves) get screwed. I believe there are some times when the scientific method should not be rigidly applied—like when people's lives are at stake.

Gosh! It is confusing trying to decide what to do about treatment and diagnosis. Presently I am in a rather large experimental program using Chinese herbal medicines to strengthen my immune system, plus acupuncture for neuropathy. I have to take 27 herbs each day. The researchers say they are working on herbs for neuropathy but don't have the mixture figured out yet. I don't know if any of these treatments are helping, but the pain is less after the acupuncture. A flu and cold are going around. Many of my friends have gotten one or the other. Since I have not gotten either one of them, I think my body is still doing fine at fighting off these buggers.

September 23—I just got home from a picnic held for women who are HIV+ along with their families and caregivers. When Marsha, our support group leader, said in June that she was thinking of having such a picnic, I wondered how many women would come to an outdoor event. Would there be a sign, "This way to the HIV+ women's picnic"? Without such a sign, how would we recognize each other? It seemed too exposed to me.

Others had the same concern, so we met indoors in a city parks building. About 75 or 100 people came. It was a very mixed group— 80 percent white, 20 percent black, with a wide range of ages, a bunch of kids, a fair number of punkers, and lots of people who looked as though they had lived a pretty tough life. A few had no teeth. It was a congenial evening. A band played for part of the evening, and some comedians entertained for about a half hour. Here are some snatches of conversation I overheard:

- "Why are you here?" [This was a code question for "Are you HIV+, or are you a caregiver?"]
- "The doctors wanted me to have an abortion, since both my husband and I were positive. This was in the early days before they knew anything. (Laughter.) When Darian was born he was negative! You just never know—and the doctors never know either. It was just somebody trying to save the world from the likes of us. What a miracle! Of course we worry about Darian when we get down. How will he grow up? Who will take care of him if something happens to us? But something will work out—it always does."
- "This AZT is really helping me. I feel better than I have in years."
- "AZT has me really down. I'm thinking about stopping treatment."
- "How's your herbal program going?"
- "First I was in an alcoholic treatment program and they kicked me out when I shared with them that I was positive. Now I've lost my job because my best friend told my boss about my status. People

are just stupid. As if I could give it to folks while selling perfume..."

I met several people who called me _____ (the name I use in registering for all HIV appointments). I said to one woman that wasn't my real name. Her response was, "Sure, probably half of the women here are here under other names. Being HIV+ gives people a chance to live beyond their own identities." Well, that's one way to think of it.

September 26, 1988—Today I did two interesting things which relate to this journal. In the early morning, I met with Ron, who called last week requesting my help with a publication on AIDS which the National Council of Churches is working on. They are writing the stories of HIV-infected people to give a face to this epidemic. They needed a woman's story. I agreed that parts of this journal might be useful for them.

Ron walked in, and right away I was comfortable with him. He had dark, intense eyes with a look around them and inside of them which I have come to associate with AIDS. I never know whether that characteristic look comes from staring into the bright light/dark that is AIDS in such a sustained and unrelenting way, or whether it results from the physical condition. Whatever, it seems to be quite common in people with infection that has advanced to the stage of AIDS.

We talked at a deep and comfortable level right away. I've noticed that this happens frequently when HIV+ people get together. A powerful bond unites us. Ron and I talked about how it had been for us and what we were learning. He had lost his job when his illness progressed to the point that he was sometimes sick. His employers confessed to feeling guilty and angry that his situation put them in such a bad position. But still they fired him, leaving him with no health insurance and no pension.

We talked about our need to admit that we were angry about what was happening in our lives. People seem to want us to go through this gracefully, but this is not always possible. Our friends who are not infected also are angry sometimes about the impact our illness has on their lives. And interestingly, sometimes they feel guilty about being on the safe shore while we flail around in the water. As for me, it is tough sometimes when it seems I cannot swim to that safe shore no matter what I do. How do we acknowledge to each other our mutual yet different angers?

This reminds me that a group of my friends who met at my birthday party got together a couple of days ago to begin educating themselves about AIDS and to explore their own issues about this epidemic. They reported that some people talked about their fear for me, others about their sadness about what I was going through, and a few were quite angry. They reported the last part as though somehow it was not okay to be angry about this shift in my reality and the effects of that change on our relationship.

Ron talked about his feelings and deep questions. He asked if I had gotten to the part of this disease where I could see the gifts it brings. I said I was not there yet, but that I could see positive aspects of some of the changes in myself that have occurred as a result of being HIV+.

Later in the day an old friend called to say that her son had just told her he was HIV+. I have known both of them for nearly 20 years. Her son had known his status for four years and was just getting around to being able to tell his parents. Of course she was worried about him. In four years he had been able to go to only two support group meetings, so frightened was he of discovery. What to say? I made an appointment to see her soon, and I will try to get a note off to him.

September 28, 1988—I called Mark to get a couple of dates I had missed in the journal entries about Dennis. I also wanted to read him the parts of this book which involved the two of them. He told me that he has a new love, but that Dennis is still very much with him. He spent yesterday cleaning out Dennis's desk. Mark needs to begin to move Dennis out of the house now.

Mark told me a story about Dennis that I want to include here, although I hoped I would not continue to add to this journal so we can go to press. Mark said that he had passed his exams to get his physician's license over the summer. He said, "You know, Dennis and I had planned to take the tests together, since both of us always had such a tough time with tests. Even when Dennis could no longer read, I would find him sitting at his desk, looking down at one of his medical texts—sometimes upside down. I would ask him what he was doing. He would reply, "I'm studying for the test."

Sometimes people think that if only they think the right thoughts or build a big enough plank into the future, they will be able to make it into that future. It doesn't always work that way.

October 14, 1988—Something happened the other day which set me to thinking. Every time one has to interface with an AIDS service agency, one is subjected to the same set of questions usually starting out with, "How do you think you got this virus?" I have noticed in conversations with AIDS caregivers that they tend to categorize HIV+ women by how they got the virus. I'm not sure why that is so important in their minds. The woman quizzing me the other day said that the AIDS virus was in the Bay Area blood pool during the time Dennis and I made love, so I could have gotten it that way. I could have gotten it through the gamma globulin shots I take each year when I go to India to do my work cleaning up the Ganges. Or, of course, I could have gotten it from the blood transfusions. I can't exactly ask the virus, "How did you get in here?" So my own situation is ambiguous.

But those of us who are hosts to this fire in our veins rarely talk to each other about how we got it, even though I suspect we spend quite a bit of time thinking about it. And when noninfected people find out we are HIV+, one of the first questions out of their mouths is, invariably, "How did you get it?" I've thought a lot about that question.

Riley, an HIV+ friend, asked Gail the other day, "Don't you think it is sadder that Fran is HIV+ than me, because she got the virus from a blood transfusion and I got it from sex?" That is a really pathetic question, and behind it is the source of much of the shame connected with this disease. This is internalized oppression. No, I don't think it is sadder. It is awful that anyone must deal with the impact on their life of being HIV+. This gives me some insight into why it is so difficult to organize all HIV+ people into a potent force in the US and in the world.

No one asked this virus into his or her life. I am convinced that most of the people with sexually transmitted viruses have not been any more indiscriminate, any wilder than many of us were when we were young. Times were pretty loose back then. Young people have sowed wild oats for generations. Judging from the scandals in the religious right, it seems that for many adults, things are still pretty loose even now. No one is really entitled to self-righteousness. There are simply some people who are paying for their wild times in very painful ways and others who are not.

Only once have I asked a friend how he got this virus. We had been riding in a bus for several hours, it was dark, we were talking "deep and real" talk. Finally I asked. He said, "You know, Fran, I just didn't think you could get it if *one time* you had sex unprotected." He is living proof that you can—and many do.

Now as to biting people. You know, it is very rare that a human bites another person hard enough to break the skin. It seems pretty unappetizing when I think about it. Generally speaking, it would be more dangerous for the biter than the "bitee." People biting others should know that if they bite an HIV+ person and get blood into their mouth, and if they have sores in their mouth, they stand a good chance of getting AIDS. So I guess one could conclude that it's best not to bite people who are sexually active with whom you do not have a trusting relationship, or persons who are IV drug users.

I have met one HIV+ woman in a support group who bit a

policeman once. I don't know much of the story. The policeman died of a heart attack while skiing. The police department pressed for a murder conviction because they claimed he died because he was so stressed out from fear of AIDS. I personally think he died because of something else; if you could die from stress of AIDS, I would have died at the end of August. And I know many others whose hearts would have stopped long ago.

It is a horrible thing for police—or for anyone—to have to worry about being bitten and getting AIDS. But it is a very rare occurrence. I don't think I have ever thought of biting anyone before this virus came into my life. Now I occasionally find it a bit humorous to think of people sitting with me, afraid I might bite them. I can't even write that without smiling. But even if I did bite you, the researchers say there is not that much virus in saliva to infect anyone. On the other hand, these surely would be hard times for Dracula.

October 26, 1988—Last night's support group was very moving, and I learned so much. One man told a story which all of us could identify with. While cutting something at a restaurant he works at, he had nicked himself and had begun bleeding on the food and on his work area. He freaked out inside, threw the food away, and went to get some bleach to clean the area. Some of his work mates asked him what he was doing with bleach, joking a bit with him about it. Of course he was not able to be open with them about why he was so careful. All day he was very conscious of the bandaid, checking it frequently to see that it was in place.

A nurse in the group reassured him, telling us how impossible it was for us to give the virus to others in this way. The virus dies very quickly outside of the body, and saliva and digestive juices would also act to kill the virus.

This opened up a long discussion about how we could feel good about ourselves when something so potentially bad is inside of us. I said I think about this every time I see my menstrual blood. This blood now seems "bad" to me. I wish I didn't feel this way; I don't think that is a good way to feel about myself. It negatively impacts my self-image on a very deep level. I think I need to change my thinking about this. But I don't know how. No great solutions emerged from the discussion, but the question is still rolling around in me. I know that I trust that man a great deal more than I did before hearing of the incident. I know how careful he is as a custodian of this virus, and how deeply he wants not to harm anyone. I feel the world would be safe in his hands. This should help each of us feel better about ourselves.

A memorable discussion centered around optimism, hope, and denial. One man accused Hal (not his real name) of being pessimistic. Hal said, "When _____ died last January it really tore me up. I had been telling him that things would be okay—sometimes I believed it and sometimes I said it because it was all I knew to say. Now I feel bad about those times I was not exactly straight with him. Things didn't work out; he is dead. I know things aren't going to be okay for me either, and I can't say anymore that they will be. It's just a matter of time."

So many people in that room had lost so many dear friends. One of the most chronically cheerful men in the room talked about how he maintains his attitude. He said, "I know I am going to be sick. And I know I am going to get well every time except the last time. There will be many getting wells before the ultimate not getting well. So I enjoy each day. I've made my peace with the down time. There is no ground that you gain and maintain. You simply find your way through your life one day at a time. And there is real joy in that."

Another man said he had told only two other people about having the "HIV disease" (that's what they are calling it now, I hear), and he felt totally unable to tell his mother. He said he would only disclose his status to her if he felt strong enough inside that he would not break down as he told her. He felt he needed to be strong enough to take care of her in her upset state.

I mentioned that my acupuncturist said my tongue was white and he had asked if I had one of the HIV-related diseases of the mouth. I didn't know much about these mouth diseases and asked if anyone had any of them, so I could compare tongues. Several of them showed me their tongues after the meeting. A few weeks earlier I had talked about the spots on my chest and whether I should get them biopsied. After that meeting several of the men in a similar fashion had taken me into a back room and showed me their posies so I could see what a posie looks like. I decided that my marks were not posies and I stopped worrying about it. This underground medicine has definite advantages in helping us to know whether or not to go to a doctor.

I told the guys about this book, reassuring them that I had kept their confidences while revealing some of what we had talked about in general terms. I felt a little nervous as I admitted that the book included parts of my early prejudices about gay sex and the gay subculture. But they eased my fears, responding that there was nothing I could say about them that they had not at one time felt about themselves. One of them said how much it meant to him that I was in the group. Tears came to my eyes as I realized how much it meant to me to be in this group with these fine people.

We talked about our commitment to each other. Would we drop out of the group if/when we got sick? So often people just vanish into their homes or hospitals and don't keep connections with friends. Maybe the group should agree to meet at the sick person's house if they were up to it. But would we be willing to have the group see us if we were not up to being our usual selves? We are not clear about this for now. I suppose it will take getting to know each other better and talking much more about this before we know what to do.

As each person spoke, I looked into their eyes and remembered what Stephen Levine said: "When people look at a glass half filled with water, some see a glass half empty, others see a glass half full. I see a glass already shattered, and the fact that it holds water is a real miracle." Knowing we have this virus is such a shattering experience that life becomes a real miracle. There is a kind of truth we can tell each other that is as precious and powerful as a holy nectar. It has the power to heal some of our woundedness.

October 27, 1988—I keep thinking I should stop this journal, but relevant things continue to happen. I talked with Chris this morning, and he told me about a vacation he and Brian took to the Grand Canyon. Neither of them had ever been there, and they have decided to do some of the things they have always wanted to do before it is too late. In describing an eight-mile hike they had taken, Chris used the term "life against stone" several times. I finally asked him what that meant.

He replied, "I saw such beautiful bright red stone everywhere. Every now and then there would be a little crack where a seed had made a home for a tree which, as it grew, split the rock open to make a bigger home. I looked very hard at that, so that when the hard times come again I will be able to remember that life lived against the stone can make a place. We can make a home for ourselves here in the stone. It's real hope, Fran."

Life does often seem to be lived against stone.

October 29, 1988—I went to check out a women's support group over at the San Francisco Aids Foundation. About ten women were in the room—ten very active street-wise women, mostly former drug addicts. Most of the women said they had been in the group several years. Two or three conversations were happening at once, as the group leader tried to keep going around the room and have each person say what was going on in her life and what good things they had to report. It was called "news and goods."

One woman's "news" was that her children were being taken away from her. Over half of the women had had some experience either with losing their children or being threatened with that loss. Another woman had put her three-year-old baby up for adoption because she was feeling so weak these days. She started to cry as she reported that they would not even let her see the baby occasionally.

A third woman defended that decision: "You have to let her go. She needs to get adjusted to her new parents without you in the picture. It will be better for her. If you love her, you will let her go. I have done it. You will get used to being without her." I was shocked that several women had partners who were also HIV+. What would it be like to live with someone who was also going through these tensions and energy swings? It seems almost impossible. But I guess it would at least be companionship.

Another—a tall and statuesque Oriental woman—had suffered from dementia but had mostly recovered. She and the group leader told me about how she had been unable to talk or participate in the group for awhile; now she really was much better. It was surprising and interesting to me that dementia is reversible. I didn't know that dementia was an up-and-down thing. I thought that once you "lost it," it was gone. The women joked about a doctor in San Francisco who gives out false AIDS diagnoses, so that people can get on the food and financial aid programs that the government and social service agencies have available. In every disaster there are those whose more self-serving instincts come to the foreground.

People referred to a member of the group, Meredith, who obviously had been an important and beloved member. She had recently died. Several times in the two hours, it almost seemed she was present in the room, the way they spoke of her.

November 1, 1988—Someone said on TV that it takes a society twenty years to learn to live with a new disease. That's what is happening in San Francisco. We are learning to live with a new disease. And the rest of the country—make that the rest of the world—is learning as well. Maybe because we are so affected by the AIDS virus here in my city, we are having a head start, a crash course in this process of adjustment. It would be so much easier if we had the words to express the images, the models, the films, and books to tell us how others have done AIDS—how they face the issues which daily present themselves at the doorstep of my consciousness. It's easy to forget in my-day-to-day living that this is new for me, new for my society, new for my own social context, and new for my species.

Bob said something the other day which impressed me. He speculated that in twenty or thirty years people with AIDS will be counted among the heroes of this time. Those heroes will include the PWAs who are the guinea pigs for the research and those who are changing sexual practices and learning to think about the society in a responsible way. If people can change something so close to their identity as their sexual practices, there is hope that we human beings can make the other changes which are essential to our prospects for survival. My friend Alan says that his greatest fear is that one day he'll be the only gay man left and he is not at all sure what he'll say about the whole epidemic.

Last night I met with some singers and performers to discuss facts about women and AIDS. I invited about eight HIV+ women to tell their stories so these performers can inform their audiences that the face of AIDS is composed of women and children as well as men, and that we all must begin to think of ourselves a little differently now.

One of the performers, a lesbian, asked incredulously, "Do you think we should get tested?"

"Is it possible you have been infected?" I asked.

"Yes," she said.

"Do you practice safe sex anyway?"

"No," she replied.

"Then the answer is 'yes.' If you are not practicing safe sex, you should find out whether you are passing on the virus."

At that moment I sensed one of the differences between HIV+ people and those who do not know their status. Most of us HIV+ folks have somewhat come to terms with our responsibility to society. At least we think about this responsibility every day. But society has for the most part not come to grips with its responsibility to itself. Instead it wants to control those of us who are HIV+ rather than find out and implement the changes necessary to protect itself.

I had another thought last night. If I had a heart attack, probably no one would give me mouth-to-mouth resuscitation these days. But from what I read, it would probably be safe. It must be tough for medical technicians and ambulance crews not to be able to tell who is HIV+.

November 7, 1988—I felt jittery all day about tomorrow's election. Never in my life have I been so personally affected by the democratic process. On my way to a meeting in the evening, I stopped by my church for some moments of calm. I stepped into the quiet sanctuary and went to my traditional seat in the second row. It was dark, the only light coming from the hallway and the moon shining through the skylight. I was surprised to look up and see polling booths which had been placed in the front of the sanctuary, since our church is one of the voting locations in the city. The cross loomed large over the polling booths. This cross in our church is made out of the burnt timbers of an earlier church which had been fire-bombed because of homophobia and hatred. My church welcomes all, but especially ministers to gay men and lesbians with the message that God loves everyone. In addition to lesbians and gays, I always add Moslems, Buudhists, Jews, Hindus, and native religious people—as well as those separated from these traditions.

It seemed ironic to sit there this evening amidst the polling booths, facing my fears about people voting tomorrow to decide whether I and my friends would have to register. The outcome would determine whether I could continue to relate freely to my doctor. I thought about the history of this country, what freedom means here, and how much this country and democracy matter to me. But as we often say in church, "we are a people mindful of our history." Sometimes very wrong things are voted in which involve life and death issues for some people. Over the long term, sanity seems to return to systems; but in the short term, some bad things do get approved by the voters. I hope this is not one of them.

I felt calmer upon leaving the sanctuary. I have done my best on this issue, and many of my friends have also worked against the initiative. We have spoken to many groups, leafletted, lobbied—we have done what is supposed to work in a democracy. Now it is in the hands and hearts of the people.

November 10, 1988—A couple of days ago the people of California went to the polls and voted against the Gann proposition that would have forced doctors to report the names of HIV+ patients, and would force HIV+ people to report their sexual contacts. They also, however, voted yes on another proposition that gives the police the right to test for the AIDS virus in anyone they arrest. Many people objected to this proposition because it is a "foot in the door" toward forced testing. I think people who voted for it did so because they feel that something must be done about prostitution. I wonder what it will take to convince those who use prostitutes to protect themselves.

I was very relieved about the Gann initiative, as were my friends. The heads of many corporations (Levi's, Wells Fargo, PG&E) came out against the initiative as did the Surgeon General. The Governor, to his eternal discredit, came out for it, which really did more to attract attention against it than anything else. The day after the election I was very tired. I could feel how defended I had been in my body. I had given talks about AIDS and the proposition and had heard some awful things from members of the audiences. (I had not, of course, identified myself as HIV+.) During the question period following one talk, a woman in the audience suggested three times that HIV+ people be tattooed in the groin area.

Friends continue to ask why I worked so hard for anonymous testing when I was going to put my name on this book. First of all, this initiative made me mad. I probably had a lot of free-floating anger from my situation anyway, but there must be a limit on prejudice. What may not harm me may still be very bad for society. There is a vast difference between me voluntarily giving you information about myself, and the state requiring that my doctor report on me. I think that if this disease drives people underground, the spread of AIDS will increase. That's the bottom line: not what will make me and my HIV+ friends comfortable, but what will decrease the swell of this epidemic. AIDS must be stopped.

Another thing about the election: throughout the campaign, the polls were steadily declaring that Proposition 102 would pass, but at the last minute over 60 percent of the voting public voted "no." I guess a lot of people made up their minds at the last minute—or the polls were wrong.

In today's paper, Dannemeyer announced that he is going to try to get this same law through Congress, and if that fails, he will place it on the California ballot again in two years. What a "blessing"!

November 12, 1988-I keep seeing, on t-shirts and stenciled on sidewalks, two sayings that refer to AIDS: "SHIT HAPPENS" and "SILENCE=DEATH."

Journal Entries
1988–1989

> *"The sun won't stop for no one."*
> —Holly Near

December 1—Gail and I had a fight. In a meeting she said, "The thing that really bothers me about this epidemic is the lack of calm. I think we should all try to keep calm." Since she was the chairperson of the meeting and no one was talking, she asked me what I was thinking.

"I feel badly that I am not able to be calm in the midst of my storm," I replied hesitantly. "It sounded a little like you were criticizing me for not having my calmness together all the time these days."

So often we "positives" sit silently in these meetings having our feelings hurt without being able to say anything, because to do so would tip our hand that we are HIV+. Who wants to do that? (I am still not too public about being HIV+.) Conversations are very tricky in situations where there are HIV+ and HIV– people because some people know who is positive and others don't. You can't talk to the person as if you know because you don't want to "blow their cover." It is like being in the underground. Social interaction and discussions are fraught with potentially explosive issues.

After the meeting, Gail told me she was angry with me for being publicly critical of her. Then she went home and I went out for coffee with other HIV+ people who had been in the meeting.

Over coffee we talked about the meeting. Another person brought up something else that had sort of bothered us in the meeting in addition to Gail's comment. One woman who is a "caregiver" (I prefer the term "carepartner," since from what I can tell the care goes both ways in most of these relationships) said, "I am learning so much from the relationship I have with Don that it is really wonderful for me. It is one of my most precious learning experiences these days. I am learning and he is dying."

I quietly said, "He is probably learning a lot from this time in his life too. Don is doing a lot more than dying just now."

Our little group stayed at the restaurant for quite awhile, hashing things over. We concluded that noninfected people may have some different realities from those of HIV+ people. It is important that HIV– people bring as much calm as they can into the AIDS world. For us too, it is a great goal. But we can't dump on ourselves because calm isn't always in our picture.

Later in the week, Gail and I finished our fight while in the car, stuck in a traffic jam. She had checked with other HIV+ people and they'd had similar reactions to her comment. We talked about how it is to be in two such different places in relation to such an important reality.

I said, "Sometimes I do feel angry that you are on a safe shore—one that I cannot swim to no matter how hard I try."

Gail responded, "Remember in the 'sixties how black people yelled at white people for being privileged? How the women yelled at the men because of their power position?" she asked. "Now I feel like a white man. When you are angry at me for something I have no personal responsibility for, it really throws me. It isn't fair and I won't put up with it! And another thing that gets to me: being in meetings with you HIV+ people is really difficult. You never say what is really on your mind. I hate it!"

I wasn't so much angry at her as at the difference in our realities. Actually, I envy her state. I am grateful to her for standing with me through all this trouble. I've got to get my anger under better control. I don't want my anger to hurt our friendship. I need friends these days—especially ones who can accept who I am and what I am going through. And Gail has surely been one of the best.

December 23, 1988—I took a break from writing in this journal while polishing the other pieces for publication, but I am very happy to get back to you. So much has happened since last I wrote.

About three weeks ago I went to my doctor and she tested my legs. She said that my right leg was slightly stronger but that the left was considerably weaker.

"I'd like to suggest you think about starting AZT now," Mimi said. "Research is showing that the sooner you start, the longer you can postpone symptoms and the longer you can live."

"Oh no, I can't believe that it is that time already. I'm not *that* sick."

"Just think about it. Maybe it would help."

"But AZT has such serious side effects. If I start now, what if, later on, it won't work when I really need it?"

"Think about it." Mimi is very patient.

"It's so expensive. Eight hundred dollars a month is too much."

"Yes, and the state won't pay for it if your T-cells are above a certain number no matter what the research shows."

I have to admit that dragging my left foot around is not a lot of fun these days, and the pain has really been getting to me. But until Mimi mentioned doing something about it, I did not consider remedying the matter. The side effects and cost were two major reasons for my unwillingness, but there was also a lot of denial mixed in. I didn't want to think I was sick enough to need a medicine. She made a good case for it, but I found myself dismissing her arguments.

The next few days were hectic, as I was producing a large benefit concert called Wings of Shelter, to fund home services and a residence for women living with AIDS. So my mind was kept pretty much off what was going on in my own life. But in a corner of my busy mind, worry about what to do about AZT was gnawing at me.

I want to mention a few things about the Wings of Shelter benefit. In June, when I began to notice that services were almost nonexistent for HIV+ women, I gathered some of my friends together and we began planning a concert which would have three goals: (1) to raise money to encourage organizations in the Bay Area to provide residential services for women; (2) to educate people that women also have AIDS; (3) to help HIV+ women know that they are not alone and that the community validates their (our) existence.

The concert was a lot of fun to produce as well as to attend. We raised some $6,000 for organizations providing housing for women with AIDS. The first show sold out, so we added a second show which was nearly full too. I recognized about 50 women who were HIV+. There were probably many I didn't recognize. It pleases me that I have come to know these women in the last six months. But most of the audience was composed of people who really didn't know that women had this virus. A safe sex kit was placed on every table of the Great American Music Hall, and a local comedian, Marga Gomez, did a really funny piece with the kits. She had everyone laughing as she got them playing with condoms, surgical latex gloves, and dental dams. Hopefully, the people at the event will remember that there are new safe sex requirements, now that they know women can also have AIDS. Throughout the evening the performers talked a little about women they knew who were living with AIDS. A great time was had by everyone I think.

After the benefit, I had to confront my decision whether to take AZT or not. A fine friend from my church came to the rescue by saying that I could have his extra AZT. He is one of the people whose doctors order extra AZT which is paid for by the insurance company. The doctor then gets it to people who can't afford this too-expensive medicine.

I called my friend David Ward, who has been grappling with this virus a lot longer than I have. He is a real expert, and it helped so much to talk things through with him. "Listen," he said, "let us take you by the hand on this. Many of us have been through this before, and we know how to do it and how AZT is. You are with experts now. The most important thing you can do right now is to take care of yourself. You'll get through this all right. We'll help you." His caring meant so much to me. I could practically feel my hand taken by the thousands who have gone before me in this epidemic. I couldn't help feeling sorry that they'd had less experienced hands to guide them.

For now I've decided not to begin the treatment. I will reevaluate this decision in a few months.

I feel confident that this virus is more harsh in this cold weather, as so many people with HIV are down these days. Probably I will feel better in New Zealand and India. I will get a new brace for the other leg which will help me feel more secure walking.

December 24, 1988—A new T-cell count revealed that my count had gained 500 points! Can you believe that?

"It must be the herbal program I'm in!" I bubbled.

Lisa replied, "No, it's you. Whatever you're doing, keep doing it. Merry Christmas!"

December 27, 1988—This week I heard the upsetting news that the head teacher of a large Buddhist community—with groups in the Bay Area as well as in Boulder and Canada—has had AIDS for three years. During that time he has been very sexually active and has not been practicing safe sex. As many as 100 people may be involved. Incredibly, he failed to inform his victims of the risk they faced having unsafe sex with him. He says he believed he could not pass the virus on, due to his "enlightenment."

Well, unfortunately, it does not seem to be working out that way. Several people who have already found out that they have the virus trace their infection directly to him. I am shocked, as are many members of his spiritual community. Their anger is mixed with pity, fear for themselves (as the group is rather incestuous), and confusion about what to do next. His board of directors doesn't seem to be able to convince him to step down as a teacher. And they are making the further mistake of trying to keep the whole thing a secret.

What a terrible thing! If he can be that oblivious to reality, that uncaring, how can we believe that any one of us couldn't? A great moral teacher committing what I would call murder. Of all the stories I have heard about AIDS, this one elicits the most shock and repulsion from everyone who hears it.

And yet, I suppose this is one of the bumps on the road to learning how to learn to live with this new disease. Everyone from every perspective has new things to learn about his or her vulnerability.

How difficult it must be to have previously thought oneself invulnerable and to have that shield so publicly punctured.

When I mentioned all this to Barbara, she told me a story that again brought home to me the dissonance of these times. Her peer supervision group of therapists had talked about AIDS last year. She had decided that whenever clients mention that they are having sex, it is important for the therapist to raise the issue of safe sex. She has been doing that with her clients ever since.

But on the personal level, she surprised herself. One night an old love from whom she had been separated for some months came on to her. She felt "so special, and so taken away by the moment," that she made love without using any protection. When her therapist asked her about it later, Barbara had to admit her foolishness. She says she really doesn't know what went through her head. It is easy to forget what one knows in the throes of passion, but when life depends upon it, it is harder to comprehend such forgetfulness.

Several friends have been reading my journal entries now, as I get ready to send the manuscript to the printer (for the first edition). Two responses particularly interested me. Several people reported that they found it tedious to read about the same upsetting subject page after page.

"Couldn't you break it up with something else? Maybe some comedy?" they asked.

"Well," I mused, "imagine how it feels to be embedded in the situation day after day. Of course being HIV+ is not all I do, and it's not even a very important part of who I am. I have my work (thank heaven), with many projects which are quite involving and interesting. And I enjoy play with many good friends. But please remember that this journal is about my experience with the new virus. I am chronicling an epidemic. As I step out of the newspaper headlines into real personhood with this virus, I may be preoccupied. Sorry about that."

A friend wrote the other day from India, as he had heard I was coming for my annual trip. He asked me to be sure that I could not spread the virus through mosquitoes before I came to their locale, as he has a wife and children to think of. Maybe they don't have good sources of information there. That's all I can figure. I wrote a paragraph reassuring them that I cannot send the virus into the world through mosquitoes. In the second paragraph I wrote:

"Now let's talk about the disease I can get from you. That disease is characterized by your fear of me and your thinking of me as a symbol of a global epidemic, rather than as your old friend. This fear threatens my health and yours, as well as society. Please see what you can do to keep this disease from spreading—especially my way, as I am very susceptible these days."

December 30, 1988—Last night I went to Hal's house for tea and a "chat." We hadn't gotten to know each other much outside of our support group. I enjoy Hal in the group a lot. We often cut up together and get to laughing outrageously about some weird thing or another.

He told me more about his lover's death and how hard it was for him. "Those months stretched me to my absolute limits. I was trying to keep my job together and be at the hospital every spare minute. I slept every night in his room. I tried to do everything I could for him. I would feel guilty when I dashed home to shower. I've been through this with all of my friendship network. Everyone is gone. I'm the only one left, and I see my number coming up someday. It is so hard to make new friends now. I don't think I will ever have friends as good as those I have lost. The old friends are the best ones."

He continued pensively, "You know, I have often thought that if it were the heterosexuals who were getting this disease, more attention would be given to a cure and to prevention. Sometimes I have actually wished for AIDS to get going in the straight communities so we could get some help with this." Hal's voice dropped and he said very seriously, "Then the other day I went to see the Quilt. I saw all those panels on the Quilt for babies who have died of AIDS. That night I lay in my bed and thought, 'I never meant that babies suffer like this! Never would I have wished this on babies. It is so terrible.' I know that my thoughts don't create reality and that I have no part of those babies getting AIDS; still I feel so bad for them."

But actually we did very little serious talking. Most of the night we spent in the kind of healing laughter I haven't done since Charlie and I stopped creating comedy material together. I really haven't ever laughed about this HIV+ stuff, and I have needed to.

Hal got the laughing started by telling about a date that he was having the next night. Since Hal's lover died, he has found it difficult to think of dating, although he does want to love again. Part of the problem is his fear that he might have to go through the death of this new love, and he is not at all sure that he has it inside of himself to do that. Another difficulty is that dating rituals have become unfamiliar to him.

Well, Hal was attracted to someone at a party the other day who clearly seemed interested in him as well. So mutual friends made the appropriate bridges and a date was set. Now Hal's fears began building in earnest. He had to face the torture of trying to decide when and how to tell his date that he was HIV+. This is such a risk! It is an agonizing aspect of dating for anyone with HIV. So Hal was relieved when the guy called him several days before the date with something on his mind.

Hal described the scene this way: "He started out, 'Hal, there is something I need to talk with you about which may affect whether you want to go out on this date with me or not. This is very difficult to bring up but please know that I will understand whatever you feel about this issue. I need to tell you something about myself and I hope you will be honest with me about how you feel. It is important to me that we start out our relationship being honest with each other. And if you are ultimately going to reject me because of this, I wish you would do it now.'

"I was relieved. I figured he was trying to tell me that he was positive. I was preparing to tell him my own situation. Imagine my surprise when he said, 'I'm a smoker'!"

Hal and I howled uproariously about that. And we told the story later on in the evening so we could enjoy it all over again.

We came up with other funny stories which fell generally into the following categories:

- first bleeding stories
- stories about getting night sweats when sleeping over with other people in their beds and feeling like you have wet the bed
- safe sex stories
- funny funeral stories
- stupid things other people have said and done to you
- stupid things you have done
- hospital and doctor stories
- looking at yourself in the mirror stories
- stories about getting the news that you were positive, and some of your early ideas and experiences

We thought about collecting these stories from PWA's and putting them on a tape called "Funny AIDS Stories." We could get the tape out for comic relief in the AIDS world. Although I've told Hal's story to several HIV– friends who did not seem to think it was so funny, every HIV+ person I've shared it with has really laughed. The tape probably would have a very select and small audience, but I think it would be a worthwhile project. We so need to laugh. Laughter is a real healer, and I felt that healing energy inside me for weeks after my evening with Hal.

January 1, 1989—Last week David Ward was not faring very well. He is having infections and is very weak. His cheeks are beginning to have dents in them since he has lost so much weight. He asked me if I could stay the night with him.

Being around very ill people has never been easy for me. And now, to be around people who are ill with the same virus I have causes the thought to cross my mind several times an hour, "Will it be like this for me? Will I have this pain and be so weak? How will I handle it if my life comes to this?" It really terrifies me. But I want to learn to rise above this self-centeredness, human as it is, so that I can help in this epidemic. And David is such a fine teacher for me. So I decided I would try an overnight with him.

During the day I drove him to the hospital for the injection treatment which he must endure every day. David told me that he needs to go on disability now. Ironically, he had just gotten a bonus for being such a good worker. But it is my impression that he is not so much a great worker in his federal job as he is a saint and a model of a real human being. He says his boss often gives him some small job to do and sends him home.

David talks to hundreds of AIDS people who call him on the phone at work for advice and encouragement. Frequently he tells them something he learned from Mother Theresa when she came here to open a house here for AIDS people: "In having this illness you have a great opportunity to allow people to express kindness that they wouldn't normally show. Have faith and don't give up hope."

I dropped David off at the hospital and ran some errands. When I returned to pick him up, I had to go into the hospital. David was lying in a bed with some clear liquid dripping into his veins. In the bed next to him was a very grey man receiving some new infusion therapy which consisted of blood dripping from a flat, round, doughnut-shaped plastic bag. I noticed that I focused my attention only on the bag—on the technology of the treatments—and not on the people.

This corner of the hospital had a number of rooms with beds and reclining chairs, filled with hollow-cheeked men getting something in their veins which they hope will save their lives "until a cure comes along." Seeing them all was even more frightening for me. "Will I be here someday? How will I afford all this?" I couldn't stop these thoughts from spinning around in my mind.

In the elevator David said, "I should stop by to see Jack who went into the hospital yesterday. His lover, Tony, was pretty broken up about it when he came by my house last night. He slept on top of me, we were both so scared. But I just can't bear to see Jack today, because I feel too shaky myself. Sometimes it is so much I just feel numb."

On our way out of the hospital we spotted another member of our church, Ron, as he slowly made his way inside for his daily treatment. He was not looking well at all. His going down is hard for both of us. We breathed a big sigh, then tried to move our attention from his fragile condition and find our way back to an upbeat path. It is not easy.

I dropped David back home and cooked us both a little lunch. Then I left for awhile as I had some other things to do. I went to a holiday party in the early evening. It was close and warm with lots of friends. I left the party a little early and returned to David's house.

David's Shanti helper, Glen, was there when I arrived. Shanti is the largest group of AIDS volunteer caregivers in San Francisco. For a year and a half since David was diagnosed with AIDS, Glen has spent several hours each week cleaning David's house, doing his laundry, and taking care of various things David might not have the energy to do. Glen welcomed me and thanked me for coming. My being there meant that he could go home and rest.

Three times during the night David awoke drenched from the sweats and called out for me to come in. I would get him in a dry cotton flannel shirt and roll him over to a dry part of the bed, rubbing his back for a few minutes to help him find his way back to sleep. His rear end has no padding anymore, and sleeping on it is painful day after day.

David is really a saint. Always gracious and kind, I have never seen him do a mean thing. The next morning as I fixed him breakfast, I mentioned how much I had appreciated him talking me through the AZT decision and what a truly fine person I think he is. His eyes filled with tears as he said, "Something good has to come from all of this. I just keep thinking that. It sometimes seems so difficult to know how anything good could possibly result from such a terrible situation, but I know we can find a way. I am trying really hard to find it." He told me how angry he is that this virus has ruined his thirties, which should have been some of his best years. Gracious and undramatic, he did not mention that AIDS had also in all probability completely stolen his forties and fifties as well.

When they build a memorial to the heroes of this plague, David's name should be prominent on it.

January 2, 1989—Last night's support group focused on some new topics. Several people talked about how hard it is to live with a person who is very sick with AIDS while knowing you are HIV+ too. Ed said his ex-lover John is in the hospital most of the time these days, getting treatment for lymphoma. John can't talk about his pain or about how hard it is for him to face the prospect of his own death. This is very hard on Ed. They had a fight about John's wanting to wear a hat to hide the fact that his hair is falling out. Evidently Ed made fun of him and is feeling very self-critical of that act, as it seems to have upset John. It is hard feeling angry at someone who is so sick, especially when that person seems to be protecting himself with pretense and denial. It must be all the harder because of Ed's own anger about being HIV+.

Phil chimed in that you have to realize that you are the most important person in your own life. He nodded in Bob's direction as he said, "Bob is sick a lot these days. I am going to have to be able to live my life even if he isn't here." Bob jerked a bit in reaction, looked a little strange, and made a heroic effort to smile encouragingly at that remark.

Phil talked about how tough the holidays were for him without alcohol and drugs. Ed says that he doesn't even have sex now and that life is hard. But mostly, he is lonely without someone to love. He never thought he would have to go through something like this alone. People nod in agreement. Someone asks if anyone else experiences frequent and consuming waves of anxiety and stress. Everyone nods.

Someone asks, "Why don't we ever mention in this group how hard the holidays are for us? Are we hitting depth yet?" Who knows? We all agree that we are afraid to get into upsetting subjects. Being raw with what we think about life, illness and death leaves us in such a vulnerable place, and we feel we can't afford to be any more depressed than we already are. It's hard to tell sometimes whether it is more depressing to talk about things or to keep quiet about them.

January 3, 1989—

NO THANK YOU!
I don't want your Christmas basket
    Damn it!
Some anonymous do-good group leaves a message
    on my answering machine
        that they would like me to have
            a Christmas basket this year.
Thanks for the charity—
    but no thanks.
    I don't want the basket
        or your pity
            because you need to find some HIV+ woman
                to fill your equal opportunity pity giving quota.
And while you're at it
    I don't want your advice
        about what stage of death and denial I'm in.
    What if I can't follow Kubler-Ross's grand plan for death?
        Does anyone get an F in death?
            Are there death underachievers?
And now that I'm on a roll...
    I don't want to be your spiritual teacher either
        or the noble exemplar "AIDS patient."

You may need me to be something I am not:
   a symbol of too much helplessness.
There's a window peeper out there
     not peering at my body
       but ogling my pain and suffering
   Getting off on my helplessness
      watching as I teeter on the high wire of HIV.
Will I get my balance after each gust of wind
   or this time fall into the net—
   or miss the net entirely and
     dash myself on the ground so far below?
      Does anybody know?
        Are you a betting man?
        What are the odds?
         Not good they say...
     99 to 100%, they say, of the people
      who drank milk as children...will die
        and it's the same odds that HIV+ folks will die of AIDS
But when....
      and under what circumstances?
       Ah! there's the rub.
I am not resigned to all this dying
   in my place
    in my time
     in my body.
This virus is not your—or my
   goddamn golden learning opportunity.
I did not choose this virus.
   I did not "create this reality"
     because somehow I felt badly
      about myself
       or my sexuality
        or because I have some "special spiritual mission."
This is a cruel and mean-spirited philosophy
invented by those who think they are sitting in the bleachers.

AIDS is a challenge to heal many wounds—
   and the strong and wise do heal
     yet this virus usually lingers.
I know you mean well
   but that's just not enough now.
AIDS means too much to everyone now.

AIDS is a terrible tornado
  a horrific wind that swoops down
    randomly picking up a trailer house
     or a whole town
      carrying it away
       crushing lives
        dashing dreams.
Does anybody see?
  Does anybody care?

We find our way
  against the wind
    or sometimes we are blown along.
We find our way
  one step at a time
    no ground gained and retained
     just one step at a time
      But we do find our way
       with help from our friends.
These friends somehow stand close enough
  to take some of the ferocity out of the wind
    as they vacuum floors and wash clothes
     for lives now too tired to do these tasks of living.
They offer a hand when weak legs need steadiness from somewhere
    drive us to hospital visits
      stay with us so we are not alone today
       hold us close when we shake and rage.
They are the calm in the eye of this storm
      and maybe even someday—
       make it a long time from now, dear God—
They will bring a Christmas basket
  when food is short
    and holidays all too precious.

Let us live in peace
  with our friends
    our chosen and accidental families
     and those close enough to know
      when we need a Christmas basket
       and when we need a swift kick in the pants.

Please let us go now
  without your pity
    or pedestal admiration
    or mindless petting.
Let us go into our lives
  nurtured by those who can help us find a place to rest
    from the burden our lives have become.

February 16, 1989—Maybe it is time to write about my time away from this journal, because it was an important time for me. I have changed quite a lot in my relationship to this virus and to myself in these recent weeks.

A "Festival of Heart Politics" was held in New Zealand. Since I wrote the book of that name, they invited me to be the keynote speaker. I plotted carefully so that no one in New Zealand would know that I was HIV+. I have been needing to get completely away from people who think of me as "an HIV+ person." I craved being in a context where people would not be worrying about me or letting me talk about it obsessively, as I have been doing more and more.

It was a rough airplane flight. We went straight through a typhoon. About one-third of the plane's passengers, myself included, deposited their dinner into the barf bags in their seats since they were too scared to get out of their seats and go to the toilets.

I arrived in Auckland at about 8 a.m. and by 9:30 I was in a meeting about my schedule. Someone from the New Zealand AIDS Foundation was there, asking if I would meet with various members of their group since I live in such an AIDS-aware city. I quietly replied that I was on vacation from the overwhelming AIDS reality in my city, but I would be willing to donate a few hours to AIDS work.

I was happy in New Zealand. I was back doing my life's work, surrounded by people who shared my interests, nestled each evening in the arms of an old friend and lover. Just to keep you up to date on my thoughts about sex and what I learned in New Zealand: I came prepared this time with gloves from the safe sex kits we handed out at the Wings of Shelter concert. I found that I did not feel stigmatized when we used them. In fact, I felt kind of heroic as we integrated putting on a glove into our lovemaking. I would say in my mind, "I am saving ——'s life right now. This is how I care for her." And for her part, she did not seem uncomfortable in the slightest.

Now a word about New Zealand. New Zealand is the kind of country it is good to know can exist. They have no nuclear weapons, and no nuclear power plants. I saw their entire Navy—four ships in the Auckland harbor. They had been invited by the British to help in the Faulkland's war, but had to decline as their entire Navy was being painted that month. Many people live there a very quiet and pleasant lifestyle—much more so than in the United States.

The Heart Politics conference was held in a rain forest, where the birds sang in the morning and people noticed. I swam in a hot and cold river where you could be warm on your front and cold on your back.

Maori people came to the conference and spoke in their own language, which was not always translated. People who knew only English sat quietly and listened without fighting. The contributions of the Maori enriched us all. One of my favorite things was when the entire group, some one hundred or so, gathered in a circle each day. For four hours they would tell each other stories, suggest ideas, or pose questions to each other. But the most wonderful part of all was that after each person spoke, in accordance with their tradition, that person would sing a song. Music definitely broke up the tendency toward intellectualizing and bull shit.

Everything went well until the last day of the five-day festival. I had been in a support group for women leaders. Each woman was supposed to take twenty minutes of group time to share her issues about being a woman leader. Now I have to admit that these days I don't find myself agonizing much about the pains of being in a leadership role. I'm sure I have the same difficulties as a leader that I have always had, but my attention and pain are in other areas. So my twenty minutes were flat and probably seemed insincere as I tried to remember what "my issues" were. The next day I apologized for being so strained. The leader said, "When are you going to talk about what is really on your mind?" I replied that I had no intention of doing that, as I was on vacation from "my stuff."

Then someone else said something which really set me off. I can't remember exactly what the triggering comment was, but I found myself in the middle of a huge and powerful wave of anger such as I have rarely felt. We were on a lake with no one around for miles, and I found myself shouting at the top of my lungs.

"You have no idea how it is to be surrounded by AIDS! I'm not going to talk about what is on my mind because I need a break. It's everywhere at home, and since I am open with my friends, they always have it in their minds that 'maybe something is wrong with Fran Peavey.' I hate it! I envy you all having normal deaths in your life from car accidents and heart attacks. You are not bombarded every week by the deaths of acquaintances and friends. AIDS is everywhere in my city once you can see it. I need a break! And I need to get back to my work. It is important to me. Once I shared what's on my mind it would pollute everything. You wouldn't really let me work, you would try to take care of me, you would worry about me. I want to go back to being the person people get irritated with when I mess up. I want people to tease me about my failings and struggle with me in a real way. I like not having to worry whether you are concerned if your children play with me. I like not having to deal with your paranoia. Being part of an epidemic is no fun—and I am having fun here!"

Blowing off all that anger was a real stride toward my own freedom. And you know, in the intervening three weeks I haven't felt as angry as I had been for months. This truth-telling may have real advantages. The other women encouraged me and were grateful for a little honesty in my sharing. Afterwards I realized how much I had needed to get far away from home. It was good for me. I intend to do this more often.

Following some time resting at a New Zealand beach, I flew to India to do my yearly consulting work with the Sankat Mochan Foundation, which works to clean up the Ganges River. What a joy it was to return to my old friends in the Foundation, and to visit the new sewage treatment "temples" that have begun working during this past year. I was delighted to see the new electric crematorium which provides complete cremation for poor people for only 50 rupees instead of the 500 it costs with wood. This means that there will no longer be half-burned bodies floating in the river. Also, over forty pink public toilets are now connected to the sewage system and they are kept beautifully clean.

When we began working eight years ago, who would have thought such progress could be made in such a short time? I have gone to consult with them about strategy every year during that time, and it is personally satisfying for me to see such change in my own lifetime. Thinking that the Indian government might not allow HIV+ people to have visas next year, and being unsure whether I would be able to come next year myself, I brought Catherine who could take my place should the need arise.

The man I work primarily with there, Mahantji, consulted his astrologer about my future. The astrologer said, "There may be a small problem with her blood, but it is not important and will be okay. She will live until age 72. Her life is not threatened." While I don't exactly believe in astrology, I really enjoyed hearing positive things being said about this body of mine which has been so surrounded inside and outside with worry and doubt about its longevity. Mahantji said, "You know, we believe in astrology. We shall not worry."

February 18, 1989—The Dark Side

As if this epidemic were not dark enough in itself, it seems important to note that a complexity of darkness is buried within the organizations which themselves bring so much light. Lest you should think that there are just these completely wonderful organizations doing fantastic things here (which is true), in the midst of this there is also disunity, competition, graft, and exploitative use of power. This is usual in any institution; to expect otherwise would be naïve indeed. Not to acknowledge this darkness might create the illusion that these errors are unseen—or worse yet, that because one is so dependent upon these institutions, one is willing to remain silent. I hope people have come to expect more than silence from me. To use the existence of this darkness as an excuse to avoid being personally involved or pressing for funding is disgusting. Darkness is a part of life and it is a part of all causes and groups.

The man under whose leadership Shanti became the great service organization it is has recently been investigated by the city government for various instances of sexism and corruption of power. He was forced out of his position. This scandal was on the front pages of the *Chronicle*, not to mention weekly fare in the gay papers for months.

There is a more difficult darkness to report. Since such good social services have been instituted here for AIDS, some people wish to take advantage of the situation. I have several times heard that a certain San Francisco doctor will give you a diagnosis paper certifying you have AIDS—even if you don't. Then you can register with all the agencies for disability funds, free food, clothes, sympathy, and transportation around the city. I wonder about these fake PWAs. What is it like for them? Are they homeless people who just recognize an easy mark? What is the doctor's motivation? Does he see himself as a Robin Hood taking from the "rich AIDS organizations" to give to the poor, or is it simply his way of making a living?

The weight of the load on caregivers causes an occasional break in the care they are able to offer. This hurts the AIDS community deeply. I heard of a doctor just losing it and shouting to a PWA, "I don't want to see you or any more AIDS patients again. Take your impossible body somewhere else!" This is an extreme case of frustration and burnout, but it hurts just the same. Increasing attention is being directed to caring for the caregivers and healing the healers. This work is vital.

Medical bills often become too great for those unable to work as much as they could in the past. Sometimes patients must cover all bills in advance and then wait months to be reimbursed by their insurance company. Others find it difficult to come up with the 20 percent they owe the doctor over what the insurance covers. It is tough for a PWA to think of changing doctors in such a vulnerable moment. Some doctors with heavy loads of AIDS cases seem to find it difficult to make ends meet without that 20 percent. It seems this conflict is handled with various degrees of grace, or lack thereof, by everyone involved.

The big picture has its dark side as well. The national response to AIDS has been shameful and disgusting—that's the only way I can put it. Several months ago, during a time in church when we were remembering yet another of our members who had succumbed to this virus, a particularly hot-headed woman jumped out of her seat, went to the front and jerked the American flag off the wall. Our confidence in our government is shattered. So many flaws in our system are exposed by the slowness of our nation and my state to recognize the AIDS problem, fund research, and find a way to provide decent care. When President Reagan declared October as AIDS awareness month in the final days of October, the insult was only exceeded by its patheticness. The presidential report on AIDS was never even accepted by the Reagan administration, let alone its recommendations implemented. So far the Bush administration has not done much better.

It is clear to me that we need a national health plan. So many have no way to pay for treatment or preventative care. We cannot allow an industry whose criterion for success is profit to be the prime mode of caring for our diseased and injured citizens.

I feel saddened by the blackness I feel inside when I think about my country and its response to this epidemic. I am reminded of the shame I felt during the Vietnamese war. This epidemic is a war involving our own people in our own land. I do not believe, as some do, that a conspiracy set this virus upon us. But I do believe there is a conspiracy, albeit an unconscious one fed by homophobia and racism, not to allocate major resources toward stopping it.

March 13, 1989—I don't feel well today. In fact, I feel terrible. My body is not doing well, and in my soul I feel so alone and wounded by I know not what except my general state and the state of our collective condition. I guess it is one of those waves of anxiety that come and go these days, without seeming to be tied to anything in particular.

I read in the paper that according to the Center for Disease Control in Atlanta, there are sufficient statistics to say that 99 percent of HIV+ people will die of AIDS or an AIDS-related disease. How can that be? Not all the people who have had the virus in the original study are even showing symptoms yet. Why do they say these things? It is really discouraging to read the paper sometimes.

So much has happened that I have not written about. But for now I just want to tell about what happened today. When I went to my acupuncture appointment, my puncturer Juan was jubilant. The last time I saw him he was also on top of the world, talking excitedly about something called ozone therapy for the immune system. Today before even saying hello, he once again started in with great enthusiasm about this therapy. He had some printed information for me about it. It seems there is a machine costing $2,000–$7,000 which makes ozone. The ozone is then put directly into the rectum. (It strikes me that there is something slightly peculiar and funny about shooting ozone into people's asses at a time when the lack of ozone in the upper stratosphere is causing global warming and threatening all of life.)

An experimental protocol has been launched in San Francisco,

Juan says. I ask who is doing it.

"Two guys who are HIV+. They are feeling much better and their T-cell counts are higher," he says.

"Are they doctors or scientists?"

"No, they are just two lovers who read the literature and found out that this therapy is being done in Germany. They decided to try it on themselves. There are so few options available that offer hope of improving the health of HIV+ people. These guys were determined to try anything they could find. They went to Germany to check it out, and now they own a machine and are doing grass-roots research. It helped them so much that they worked out a deal with a university to do a test under their auspices."

Juan's eyes sparkled as he told me, "Their T-cells zoomed upward under this treatment. It is the only thing besides herbs which I have ever heard of that makes any sense to me! It's non-toxic and non-invasive. It superoxygenates the system. And it slows down aging too!"

Juan has been HIV+ for about ten years. "It's time for me to do something," he says with a foreboding tone. "I don't keep track of things like my T-cells or stuff like that, but I can feel it is getting to the time when I have to do something. If this works we can set up these machines in basements in each neighborhood. We can really help people. The only real cost is the purchase of the machines. But wouldn't you know it. There is a move underway to require a license for ozone manufacture, and if that is enacted, making your own ozone would require a prescription. If they do that, we'll just make our own. We will do it underground."

March 15, 1989—The other day I was at Cliff's Hardware Store on Castro Street when a fire truck pulled up in response to an alarm. As the firemen jumped out of the truck, they were pulling on latex gloves before their feet hit the street. I had to laugh out loud. How crazy the world it! I support the firemen needing protection, but wouldn't you think they would wait until they saw blood to put on their gloves?

March 16, 1989—The National Council of Churches came to town last week to review and deliberate about their AIDS policy and get a publication ready. First they came to our church. About sixty members of their delegation walked hesitatingly into our sanctuary. Panels from the Quilt lined the wall.

The AIDS healing service is very popular. It is an upbeat service and the spiritual struggle and victories are palpable, even though illness and disability are also obvious. All the people doing the service were HIV+. The sermon was given by Ron, who was fired from his position as pastor of a church in Seattle with no disability when he became sick.

I read a scripture. Then we did our traditional AIDS healing service. In AIDS healing we do not necessarily think of healing as being synonymous with being "cured." Anyone from the congregation who wishes to receive the suffering and cares of people goes to the front. They form groups and one at a time—or sometimes in family or friendship units—people come up to share their concerns and be prayed with. Usually four or five little groups gather in front, with a waiting line. People often pray for healing of their fear, anger, and uncontrolled grieving.

"I just got my T-cell count and it has dropped 100 points. I feel so scared and I don't know what to do," someone might say.

Or sometimes friends pray together. "We are having a hard time with commitment since Gary has found out he is HIV+. He is afraid to let me close to him, and I am afraid that his situation will take over my life. We love each other very much but need help with the impact AIDS is having on our relationship."

I once asked for help with the sense of shame I was feeling about having HIV. It is very moving to see people bringing this deeply wounded part of themselves into the presence of God and friends with trust that others can touch these deep hurts and tenuous lives with love, care, prayer, and the power of connection.

The next day six of us from the church went to talk to the National Council's commission which is working on an AIDS publication to influence church policies. Most of them had previously met only one person who was HIV+: Ron, who has been on the commission for quite awhile.

We talked to them about how the marginalization of gay people and IV drug users threatens intelligent AIDS policy decisions in this country. We shared how difficult it is to carry on at the front line of this struggle. I debated about whether to disclose my HIV status to them. Finally, I did. I wanted them to have another face (and a woman's face at that) to attach to the headlines which seem so abstract to them.

Many commission members spoke about how filled with life they felt in our worship service. Others said it had been a peak worship experience for them.

One person said that we were a "church-dividing issue." How much more abstract—and insulting—can one get? I don't know what kind of skill it must take to go from real live people to thinking about these people only in terms of "issues," but I don't consider this a pro-survival talent. I was personally offended by being called an issue. But they did seem to get the sense of life and joy that we have together as we struggle in community about the meaning of life, death, and suffering.

April 3, 1989—While I was in the midwest on a comedy performing tour, I noticed a book on the shelf of a professor I was visiting. The title was *Divine Hunger*. I had just been thinking about what "spirituality" was for me, and in particular why my faith in God has not been challenged by AIDS. Sometimes I have wondered if I don't have a deep enough faith or if maybe I don't think about it enough, since so many people around me find the AIDS epidemic challenges their belief in God.

In my own personal history, the mountains, rivers, trees, and land of Idaho were my first and truest spiritual home. When I "discovered" God in college as I looked into a microscope, I could begin to perceive the awesome complexity of creation. I knew I was a tiny part of that whole magnificent and intricate system.

It seemed at the time, and still does, that my place in that system was to love responsibly all of life—myself, my neighbors, and the rivers, mountains, and trees. To me, God is not particularly a single being or a personal God, although I feel an intensely personal relationship present to God in my own way. I am not going to discuss here who Jesus, Moses, Mohammed, and Buddha were, or anything like that, but I do love these great teachers of our species. Due to my cultural background and personal history I probably have a greater love and respect for Jesus and Moses—but I think this is mostly because of familiarity.

I experience God in the beauty and general benevolence of all nature. When nature turns against us and becomes a tornado or an earthquake—or AIDS—God is found in the joke, the tears, and the love that heals us and allows us to go on. For now, for me, there is life and motion in all atoms—inside of me, outside of me, and in all the stars. That motion is essential to life. The benevolent part of motion in nature can be called God or whatever you want to call it. This is the key to life. In all of God and in all nature is the desire that I, and all people, animals, and plants, have good lives and respect and cooperate with the life forces on earth. This is my faith.

This does not mean that death is an evil I fight against. Death is a part of life. Life is always in death, just as death is always in life. It seems both logical and borne out in my personal experience that some aspects of the self continue to exist after the death of the body. Earlier in my life when I was quite ill, I felt myself resting in the hand of God and knew that there was a lot more to life than I had ever known before. I shall cooperate and promote life, but not against death.

Evil is the promotion of death, whether it be in war, in toxic chemical spills, or in humiliating other people and not honoring the dignity in each individual. Evil is drugs that harm life...oh, I could go on, but I am getting bored with this listing of evil. In my view, evil exists in greater complexity than I can go into here. It is not a code coming down from the past, rather it is operational in its effects on life and is most often born of the oppression and suffering on the part of the person(s) who is creating the evil. Violence against all forms of life surrounds us, giving rise to fear and deceit. One of life's great purposes is to confront that fear, oppresion, and suffering—inside of us and outside of us—and work to change it. The more I work to change things, the more I realize that I have no idea of what is the best way to do that. Still, it seems to me that there are clearly some things not to do. One is to lie to myself. Another is to do nothing about what I know.

God is found in all of life. To love God is to love life. Embedded in all life is that part of God which longs for life to continue. I experience a deep hunger inside myself which is the hunger of that part of God in me longing to drink of God in other people, animals and nature. I sense this hunger when I am terribly busy, emotionally shut down, out of touch. I think many Americans experience a similar hunger either consciously or unconsciously. Happiness arises when the hunger of the little piece of God inside of me is filled. That hunger is satisfied when I communicate with that of God inside of me, or when I am in deep communication with that of God in the life all around me.

Anyway I was so grateful to find a book about this direction of spirituality, *Divine Hunger*, that I asked to borrow the book. What a disappointment to find this book was an academic defense of cannibalism! Still, it was interesting to read. I learned that cannibals don't have the sense that they are being abandoned by their loved ones who die. By eating the dead, cannibals believe their loved ones remain with them forever.

April 4—I returned to San Francisco to find that a friend, Jim, had committed suicide by jumping out of a four-story building. He had only told two people outside his support group about being diagnosed with AIDS. His best friend told Jim's boss about Jim's illness and as a result Jim was fired. Jim could not stand to live in that world of suspicion, in which trust had become so impossible for him. So he chose to die now rather than later.

Another friend asked me if this would be considered an AIDS death. There are many suicides in the AIDS world. I don't know if the officials label these as AIDS deaths, but I do. I consider Jim's death to have been caused by the socially transmitted disease of distrust and fear. I feel outraged at the evil which took Jim from this world.

We discussed suicide in our support group when I got back. Everyone was shaken by Jim's death, as he was healthier than many.

Ken is having lots of neurological troubles these days. Sometimes without any warning his hand grips up and won't work. Other times his tongue feels heavy and sluggish. His memory for short-term details and appointments is noticeably weaker. And he is having trouble with his eyes. He is afraid he will not be able to drive his motorcycle anymore. How will he get around? He lives on top of a hill where there isn't good bus service.

One of Ken's closest friends lived curled up in a fetal position for almost a year. The virus had attacked his nervous system. Ken doesn't want that to happen to him. He has a gun. It gives him comfort to have some control of this uncontrollable life. He doesn't want to die by inches. He talks about how humiliated he often feels, and about how surprised he is that his life is going this way.

The lively discussion indicates that everyone has done a lot of thinking about this subject. Gene, a 20-year-old Latino, says he tried numerous times to kill himself when he was young, but now he very much wants to live. And now he has to deal with AIDS! He intends to fight hard to stay alive.

I say that I think we should be merciful to ourselves when life becomes impossible. Throughout my life I have taken good care of the life God has given me. I brush my teeth, wear seatbelts, don't take meaningless risks. I would never blow away a life that was really possible but I intend to be compassionate with myself when, in my judgement, too little life is left in me to make living meaningful. I intend to consult with friends and have them with me—but I shall not passively wait for the virus to take me by inches. This is a controversial position and everyone wonders if they would really be able to do it when the moment came. Me too. It is a good-humored discussion, but heavy.

Someone mentions that another HIV+ acquaintance was run over by a truck the other day. I earnestly observe, "We had better watch out for trucks these days." Laughter fills the room. We're watching out for so many things that could kill us. Our time together ends with a brief debate about whether we still believe in a good and merciful God.

April 7—I got a letter from a friend which interested me. She reported on a speech by J. Alfred Smith, who she says is among the most highly regarded black preachers in America today. She wrote:

"The heart of his presentation turned out to be about AIDS, to my surprise and delight. He told a story about a friend of his in Oakland, a medical doctor, who asked Rev. Smith to bring two other ministers to his church so the doctor could speak to them. A meeting was arranged.

When they came together, the doctor came right to the point: "I am tired of doing your work. My patients have AIDS. And I am weary. I cannot pray for them, listen to their anguish, *and* attend to their medical needs all by myself. I am tired of doing your work." And then he told them, "People in your churches have died of AIDS. But you didn't know they died of AIDS. And you didn't know because they didn't feel they could tell you."

Rev. Smith's church has created an AIDS task force that seeks to provide comprehensive services to people with AIDS. They believe that the church is about loving people regardless of who they are. The church is to be inclusive—Jesus would have wanted it that way. Anyone who has AIDS is a child of God.

He continued, "The truth is, I'm a soft person. I talk tough, but I'm tender-hearted. I can go to visit an AIDS patient one day. But I can't go the next. I break down and cry. I cry all day. I have never been as touched by anything as I have been by this. I decided I must help get this message out."

This is really important because the largest growth in AIDS is currently among Black and Latino people, and Asians are being hit too. Women are also increasingly affected. And women on the average only live 45 days after being diagnosed with AIDS because of the poor medical care, the secrecy and lack of community support. Unless these communities take the threat seriously, they will experience losses comparable to what the gay men's community has faced.

April 10, 1989—Yesterday I did a comedy show in Santa Barbara. I announced to the audience that I had written a book about AIDS which was for sale in the lobby.

After the show, a man came up to speak with me. After waiting until everyone else had left he told me he has AIDS. I looked closely at him. I could see the telltale signs: thin, bluish-purple marks on his neck and arm. He said he didn't know how to go on. "How do you find your way?" he asked me. It wasn't an easy question.

As we talked further, it came out that he was homeless and had lost his job and "lady friend" after being diagnosed with AIDS. So he left and went on the road in search of a better place to live. It looked as if it had been awhile since he had bathed or put on clean clothes. I wondered to myself how it would be to be sick and not have a warm home to retire to when the sweats came, when he needed just to rest in quiet.

Several times the question came up again, "How do you keep going?" I mentioned to him about support groups, meditation, making room for my fear and accepting it, allowing myself to grieve the losses. I passed on the most encouraging words I could remember from Gail, David Ward, Jill, and so many others. I tried to talk a little about what I have learned from my church about healing from the suffering we have in our relationship with life.

Then I asked him how he keeps going. He looked back at me with a vacant stare and said, "I'm not sure I am going. I can't really tell anymore. It's hard, very hard." All I could do was nod and touch his hand in solidarity.

He hung around, chatting with me and helping me pack my props. I asked him if there were many in the homeless community who had AIDS. "Oh sure. I've met some," he replied almost casually.

When I returned to San Francisco, the *Bay Area Reporter* had some shocking statistics on this very point. According to Rev. Donald Jackson, superintendent of the San Francisco Rescue Mission, there are between 350 and 650 homeless people with AIDS in San Francisco (depending on whose statistics you believe). At least that many additional people have ARC and are too sick mentally and/or physically to work or cope with the welfare bureaucracy.

Thinking about homeless people always gives me a hollow feeling in the pit of my stomach. But compounding being homeless and having AIDS seems just too horrible to imagine. I know we can do better as a nation and as a species regarding the people involved in both of these tragedies.

April 19—While having a massage yesterday, my masseuse, Terry, evidently dislodged a small pimple on my head. When she reported that some liquid came out, a ripple of panic passed through me. She seemed unworried, but I insisted that she go wash her hands thoroughly and avoid that area entirely. Since that fateful day nearly a year ago when I found out I was HIV+, I have felt a part of myself constantly standing guard against hurting any other person with "my bodily fluids."

An incident recently occurred that showed me how much on guard I have become. A few weeks ago Kim, a business colleague of mine, and I were in Vietnam working on some television shows. As we rode through Hanoi in a car, a truck came barrelling down on us from a side street and we were almost in an accident. I immediately thought to myself, "What would Kim have done if I had been hurt in that accident?" I pictured myself bleeding, having someone reach in to stop the bleeding or apply a bandage or move me, getting blood on them. I would be surprised if ambulance people wear gloves in Vietnam. Would he warn them, thus slowing my care and making it nearly impossible to stop my bleeding until we got to the hospital?

This virus not only attacks our bodies, it dramatically affects our sense of ourselves and our relationship to others around us. In a single moment when the nurse says those fateful words "You're

HIV+," your life is changed. I no longer felt I was me. I had become something I did not comprehend—someone I did not know. I had to get acquainted with this new self and its responses and responsibilities very quickly. Life (mine and others') depended upon it.

Being HIV+ is being vulnerable all the time. Along with vulnerability through the possibility of harming another, as the T-cells drop one is vulnerable to the bugs of others. I just finished a bout with pneumonia. Sharon tells me that I should be careful of being close to runny-nosed children and adults for awhile.

Finding out one is carrying a deadly virus—deadly to the self and deadly to those one loves intimately—is a real assault on the whole organism's sense of itself. It is devastating to find out that one is home to a deadly virus that wanders around everywhere in the body, posing a threat to the bodies of other people if it gets out. It is especially hard to learn that it is most likely that I could pass this virus either to someone who was trying to help me medically, to someone who was loving me sexually, or to a baby I might birth. This is a painful triple vulnerability. Its meaning is complex for me. It is difficult even to find the words to talk about it.

Through my involvement in the women's movement, Judy Chicago's art, and my own inner work, I had managed to leave behind the notion I got from my parents and society that my genitals were dirty and unacceptable. Now finding that that part of myself—my genitals, freshly integrated into my positive view of myself—was the place through which the virus was most available, was—well, this was a crushing blow to my positive sense of those dear genitals. I turned the whole thing over and over in my mind. A new repulsion arose. I stopped being able to touch myself there. As if to tease me, I developed an itch in the genitals which was part of some vaginal infection common to HIV+ women. The inner battle became excruciating.

Then to my delight, I found a little rock to stand on amid the rapids. I heard that women's genitals only become flooded with virus when sexually excited. I was quite happy with this boost to my self-concept. This newly gained ground was quickly lost when Jill pointed out that the only time anyone else besides me would be down there anyway would be an exciting time.

Eventually I hit upon another idea. "I am the only person in the entire world who can touch myself there safely," I thought to myself. In one way it makes me kind of special, but in another way it is sickening.

I have found it tough to integrate the idea of a dangerous virus into my sense of a fully whole and safe self. Finding a way to feel good about myself as a sexually functioning, proudly safe, and joyously orgasmic woman has been even more difficult. Somehow I intend to heal these wounds and find my way to that higher ground. But I don't pretend to be there yet.

April 20—I have had several very deep talks with Chris recently. We've been having lots of "business meetings" at which we usually transact about fifteen minutes of business and then spend another several hours talking about the real business of life.

I see a kind of desperation in him as he wrestles with a variety of concerns. He wonders how he can stop the full life he lives taking care of everybody else, so he and Brian can travel and be together now while they are still able to enjoy these things. He is the key leader in an AIDS organization and has been immersed in negotiations for better treatment for AIDS people. Many people in the community also look to Chris for advice and help regarding business concerns. So he is constantly busy. He sees time ticking away in his own life. His great fear is that he might end up sick with none of his dreams fulfilled. He and Brian want to go to Spain. They also hope to get a place on the river and spend some extended time together.

Chris confided to me that his memory is not as good as he thinks it should be. He spends a lot of time staring out the window at people on the street below his house, wondering and worrying about all kinds of things—or wondering about nothing. He has lost so many friends that I think he is in some kind of prolonged shock.

One of our recent talks was so deep and wise that finally I had to ask if I could record it. He agreed. Listening to the talk again, I am struck by how often he says, "We have to keep focused on the important things of life." To him this means talking in a real way to people and helping each person he can through this trying time. He spends countless hours with people on the phone who call him up just to help them keep going. He keeps trying "to make sense of it all."

"You know Fran, I knew Patient Zero," he said slowly. "Intimately. I looked at his picture in the paper once and thought to myself, 'That's where I got it.' I was in the first level of those infected. You know, he was a really fun person too," Chris added with a smile.

Patient Zero is the flight attendant who is supposed to have first brought AIDS from Africa. They say that because he traveled so much, he got the virus going in several gay communities. Chris has to live with the probability that he was unwittingly the route of transmission to others—possibly including Brian. We don't talk about that guilt. It hangs in the air, but I can't bring myself to open that wound and expose both of us to the pain of it.

I've heard several people share their feelings about the activities they were involved in during the early days of this epidemic, while they were trying to decide the validity of emerging information about the necessity of safe sex practices. Of course, most people did not immediately start practicing safe sex when they first heard about the possibility of some virus—or gay cancer—roaming around the gay community. It took some convincing. Now some people blame themselves for not changing their sexual practices sooner, as it might have saved lives.

"But," Chris says to me, "you know, if I had a choice—to live as an openly gay man and ultimately have to know the pain that is AIDS, or to live pretending to be a straight man but be spared the anguish of AIDS—I would choose my life all over again. I've lived and loved with integrity. I've had a good and honest life. I've been who I am and had a good time. I have no regrets—well, maybe a few, but not about the most important things."

We start plotting how he and Brian can get a place in the country and get more time together very soon.

April 25, 1989—I had an upsetting conversation with Dora, a new friend who is HIV+. I met Dora at a political meeting having to do with protesting the time it takes for new drugs to be tested. She is moving back to North Carolina soon to live with her family.

We talked about intimacy. She told me about how relationships have been for her after finding out that she is HIV+. Dora has noticed that some women moved close to her in a rather strange way. Now that she looks back at it from a distance, it seems to her that their drive to be sexual with her was more out of their need to make her happy than anything else. They so feared that they would not be up to the task of being her friend that they drove in very close rather than take the slow path toward intimacy and sexuality. An active element of deceptiveness was also involved, in that they did not tell her that they were really committed to someone else. She speculated that they were afraid they would not be up to the challenge of "loving someone with such a tough life," so they moved in very close. It's possible that they were lying to themselves and surely lying to her about their other relationships.

Dora's eyes became moist as she told me about how hard those rejections were. She has given up on the idea of ever loving someone deeply again. "It's the little deaths of your dreams that are the toughest," she said. "It's not that I want someone who would stay with me through all the really bad times. That would be nice, but I think my family will be able to do that. But until those times come, I really wish I had someone to love. I have so much love inside, and I wish I could give it to someone. Not having someone love me is not as hard as having no one to love. So I am going home."

What she said struck a deep chord in me. I told her I have been having similar experiences in my intimate life. When I first started performing comedy, people used to think they loved me and would come on to me. I could easily spot these inappropriate advances and deal with them. I sense a similar element of blindness and inappropriateness in some of the advances I have experienced in this last year. In one instance after considerable loving, the woman simply said, "I am not sure I could deal with you dying. I don't think I am up to that." That really hurt deep inside. What could I say? I'm not sure I am up to it either. And I am relatively sure I will not do it perfectly. But to stop living and loving now because of what might be down the road seems to put me at a real disadvantage in finding someone to love. I am not ready to give up on loving yet, but I can understand Dora's letting go of that which no longer seems possible for her.

Dora said that she has never met anyone who was HIV+ who had formed a loving relationship after knowing that they were positive, except for a few men who formed relationships with other HIV+ men. I asked around and none of my friends knew anyone either. This has started me looking for people who know something about being HIV+ and forming new relationships. Lots of people have dreamy advice to give in this area. To me their comments sound more like Snow White than the real world. There is little really sound advice about how to handle the issues that come up in our situations.

I'm not ready to face this "little death." Just now I am feeling a lot of hopelessness about it.

April 27—Talks with Chris have intensified these last few days. Although we get together to discuss business, our attention soon turns to other things. A few days ago he started the conversation with the news that his T-cell count has dropped to around 325. Also this week, Brian has found what looks like the first lesion on his body. He says they have both been very upset for several days.

"I have to start doing something about my health now—probably including starting AZT," he says. "And more than anything I need to cry. But it is hard for me. Maybe I will go to see my minister. She is someone I could cry with."

Several days later I saw him again, and the tension was visible on his face. "Still no crying," he reported.

During last night's talk with him I inquired once again about how his crying was going. He said the dam finally broke on Friday. His friend Bob died early that morning, and he went over to Bob's house to get rid of the hospital bed and pills so that Bob's parents wouldn't have to deal with that.

Bob had been very sick these last two years—"sicker than most, and for longer," Chris reported. Bob's formerly homophobic parents had come out from Texas and ended up spending the last two years not only taking care of Bob, but helping all the "other boys" in Presbyterian Hospital as well. Bob's mother was known as "Mom" to AIDS people all over the city because of the many kindnesses she shared with them—making cookies, listening, sitting with them at their bedsides, running errands. Now she talks about how she will miss not only Bob, but all of "her boys" when she goes back home. She says she will help take care of the AIDS people in Texas because "they don't have any community care system like we do here."

Bob's funeral is on Saturday. Sunday is Mother's Day, and Chris and a bunch of "her boys" are taking "Mom" out for the day. I marvel at the changes this epidemic brings to so many relationships. Something good *is* coming from all this—it's hard to see it, but occasionally we do feel positive elements in the midst of all this suffering. New ways of caring, of being together beyond old boundaries of thought, age, and prejudice are emerging. Minds and hearts are not permanently locked.

So Chris got to cry for Bob, for himself, and for all the accumulated experiences of suffering in the shadow of this epidemic. Sometimes people report that they have lost so many friends that they no longer find it possible to cry.

May 1—Today Allan and I were talking. He is still in touch with an old lover from high school, Jeff. Jeff is now married to Marsha but has continued to have occasional sex with Allan. Allan swears that they have had only safe sex since AIDS hit our community. Marsha, Jeff, and Allan are close friends and do many social activities together.

A few months ago Allan was diagnosed with AIDS and he told Jeff. Jeff immediately freaked out. "Don't tell Marsha! She will kill you!" (A classic case of projection, wouldn't you say?) He refuses to get tested and keeps calling Allan with all kinds of paranoid thoughts that people are trying to kill Allan. It's no wonder that Jeff is feeling paranoid. Think of all the blocks in communication and real connection between these old friends, stemming from his denial and secrecy.

Allan is very embarrassed about his feelings of shame, fear of reprisal, and guilt. We need a new word for this sense of having done something that turns out to have harmful consequences. Guilt isn't exactly the right word.

May 9—Sue said to me the other day, "After reading your book, I realize I know a lot about how HIV feels. But what actually happens inside the body?" I had to chuckle. Ever since my first visit with Lisa when she asked me if I wanted to know what to watch for with this virus, I have tried to keep my mind off my increasing awareness of what AIDS means. Of course it is impossible to do this. One hears every day, "Harold is back in the hospital and is very confused. He is on mask oxygen and not doing well." "John is not able to go out now—he can only stay in his bed. His legs don't work anymore and neither does his brain, really."

AIDS is a terrible death. AIDS is a long, painful, and humiliating death. Prior to that there are months and years of fevers, random infections, skin rashes, shingles, diarrhea, neurological disturbances such as hands going out, tongues not working, infections in the mouth and genital areas, legs hurting, heart infections, random sweating, shortness of breath, short-term memory loss, weight loss, blindness, long-term memory loss, pneumocystis pneumonia, lesions all over the body but particularly disfiguring on the face, muscles eaten up, herpes, and in general infections and pain everywhere. It's not a pretty picture.

It is understandable that HIV+ people anxiously focus their attention on every little pain and problem. Faced with this experience, it is especially annoying when drugs on trial in one's own city or legal in another country for treatment of AIDS are still unavailable to people on their death bed.

May 10—I just got off the phone with Chris. It was a very interesting talk—on many levels all at once.

His Beta count is up, so for sure he is going to start AZT now. "You know," he said, "we are running a foot race now, and it is a race we all want to finish last."

Lately he has been realizing how little he has understood what Brian has been going through this last year on AZT. Now that he is facing the same situation, Chris is critical of himself for not having empathized more with Brian. "Now that I feel myself sliding into the world of the untouchables—into the world of the ill, where the characteristics of the ill are becoming my own characteristics—I wish I had been kinder to those who I saw go before me. As Bob slipped away, I did what I could, but I did not gleefully include him in my life. Now I can see people leaving me behind when I can't keep up with them. The trick is to be forgiving of those people who are leaving me behind—and to be forgiving of myself for having done to my dear friends what my friends are now doing to me. I'm not sure I know how to be that forgiving yet, but I hope I learn quickly."

Chris switches topics and tells me he is feeling quite optimistic about compound Q, a substance derived from cucumbers. He has heard a rumor that this medicine was tested at the university on HIV+ people without FDA permission, and that it was very effective.

"The results are hopeful," Chris says enthusiastically. "It actually kills the virus even in the macrophages."

I say, "Even in the macrophages?!" I don't really know what macrophages are, but it is one of the many special HIV words that have entered my language. All I know is that we want to keep the virus out of the macrophages, wherever they are. "Wouldn't it be ironic if the cure for AIDS is found in an ordinary cucumber?"

Anyway, after obtaining such positive results, the researchers then went to the FDA and demanded that the 18-month waiting period be waived, or they would go public with their results. "If that happened, there would be rioting in the streets. No one would put up with these stupid waiting regulations anymore. So the FDA evidently relented. This is not like psoriasis, where 18 months isn't a matter of life and death."

It seems that some researchers are evidently taking a proactive position for us with the FDA. They are learning to play politics and doing it well. It's about time! It's encouraging to us that there are people taking real risks to get things moving. Chris and I spend a few minutes trying to think of how to express our gratitude to these people.

"Sometimes it is difficult to remember on how vast a scale all this suffering is happening. Life almost gets to seem normal, in a bizarre kind of way. We adapt to each new change as if it is only us involved. But when I think about people all over the country—all over the world—going through this, it is really appalling. Things just seem to be going along as usual for so many people. But you are going to a funeral tonight and I am going to Bob's memorial on Saturday. We remember. Do you recall the times when we didn't have funerals to go to every week or so? And when we feel things in our body, it gets harder to forget. Gosh, this is a strange life we are living!"

Then we go through the now familiar loop of "Do we really think a cure will be found or not?" I tell him I don't expect a cure, because this is a retrovirus, and they have never found a cure for a retrovirus. My hope is that they will find a way for us to live with the virus in an inactive state until we die of old age. Chris responds, "That will be good enough for me, but frankly, I'd like a cure."

On another track, Chris tells me that he was recently involved in an automobile accident. He got out of his BMW to find its front all crushed in. While talking to one of the spectators, the guy commented that Chris was remarkably calm and good-natured about the whole thing. Chris said to him, "When you've been dealing with AIDS for over a year, this kind of thing doesn't really seem very important. What's a crushed BMW in the whole scheme of life?" He continued, "I figured that I would never see him again. Why not just tell him the truth about what I was thinking, rather than guard against the truth coming out? Just for once. It felt quite liberating."

Of course, during our talk another track keeps weaving in and out of the conversation: the business matter which was the excuse for the phone call in the first place. We keep returning to business every few minutes because we have to make certain decisions.

"Now, back to more mundane matters," Chris says, "When should we close this escrow?"

"As soon as possible," I say.

"Yes, we should do everything as soon as possible," he agrees.

May 14, 1989—Today, one year after my visit to the clinic to get my test results, I went to consult with the fig tree in my back yard. Even this week I am in the process of moving to another home, so there was a bit of a farewell in our conversation.

I reviewed this past year and thanked the fig tree (standing in for all of nature) for its steadfastness. I tried to summarize my year's journey along this HIV path:

- I am happily back working internationally. I have done rewarding work in India, New Zealand, and Vietnam as well as touring the U.S. Traveling is still intimidating for me, especially when I go to places with little HIV experience. Over and over, I go through inner loops of fear followed by recommitment to remember what I am doing with my life. In spite of my fears that I might run into prejudice in the homes where I stayed, fortunately I did not. And more significantly, I did not let my fear of that prejudice stop me from doing my work as usual. I am always happy for a chance to get away from the cauldron that is San Francisco these days. But when I come back, the news of my friends is rarely good.

- I feel mostly back to normal except for the occasional blip of confusion and illness on my screen. I have had a few small illnesses, including one light case of pneumonia (not pneumocystis pneumonia), and I did not die of fright. My legs continue to cause me trouble but it is not a steady decline and both the pain and dysfunction are somewhat variable. I continue to be a part of a Chinese herbal research program for HIV+ people. We take 27 herbs each day. I also continue doing envisioning work during my morning meditation period. I concentrate on sending the virus out of my body. "If I die so do you," I tell the virus, "so may I suggest you just go down to the kidney and out in my urine. That's the way out." I see these little gremlins jumping out of my blood and into the kidney tubes. "And if you can't get out yet, keep moving. Don't stop anywhere. In transit—that's the way for a good virus to be." I don't know if it helps them find their way out of my body, but I find an inner satisfaction to the envisioning, so I do it.

- I am in a new support group and hope to join a dance class soon for people with HIV disease. I want to teach my feet that they are dancing feet instead of stumbling feet.
- My social network has really learned how to be supportive, and not only for me. Many of my friends are now volunteering in one way or another for HIV+ people. I have learned to be more open with my friends although I still go through occasional loops of secrecy.
- Friends have pulled together a medical fund through a tax deductible foundation to help with my medical bills. It was organized by another HIV+ woman in my social network who does not have problems in financing her own medical care. Her compassion and empathic support have really moved me.
- I am learning to make time for friends and leave that time uncluttered so that we can really communicate. I have put more energy into resolving long-standing conflicts in my life. I have become much shyer about going to social events but occasionally these last few months have ventured forth and have not felt too different.
- Things seem okay with my family although I sometimes feel farther away from them these days. I have no way of knowing if they would come through for me if things got really tough. This not knowing adds a level of insecurity to my alternatives in the future. I am sure reading this book will pose some surprises for them.
- I continue to puzzle about the presence and form of the love in my life and what effect my virus status has on my intimate relations. I find commitment more complex. And I note some aspects of the love people offer seem more attached to my illness than I wish. Never very adept in the area of intimacy, I am moving slowly. But safe sex is not unmanageable for me, and I no longer feel so stigmatized by the necessity of it in my new life.
- More services have become available for HIV+ women during the past year. A house for women PWA's and their children has opened, and several more are in the planning stage. I hear a support group for non-drug-addicted HIV+ women is going to start soon. Friends tell me that more women are in the AIDS ward of the hospital these days.
- I notice subtle changes in my life. I try to stay out of the sun and wear good sunglasses, as the researchers say that ultraviolet light multiplies the virus very quickly. I am moving into a new house which is all on one level and has a level garden, so I can continue my hobby of gardening without stumbling. It is less expensive so my monthly expenses are lower. Unfortunately I

had to leave my fig tree at the other house, but I plan to plant another soon.

With all these adjustments, some balance seems to be returning to my life. I have started taking the newspaper again. No longer do I read every AIDS article and fuss about each little fact and statistic.

A slight breeze of optimism and hope permeates the AIDS community these days. It comes from new therapies, from people living longer, and from the evaporation of some of the social pressure we feel from the threat of repressive legislation. These signs are very real yet breathtakingly fragile. A countervailing wind is the continuing death among friends. This is a war zone. But some people are feeling the possibility of a treaty in the foreseeable future.

I have come to love a lot of new people, many of whom are fragile and living tough lives. Sometimes I find little ways of helping. I get satisfaction in knowing that I can be part of the community as a partner—not just part of the problem. More and more I come to value the wisdom found in PWAs, and in other people who have found a way to stand calmly with us.

I constantly wish David Ward could teach people what he has learned about loving people and letting people love him during these last several years. He is an expert who can share not only about what it is like living with AIDS, but also lessons from AIDS which apply to all the human dilemmas we face. The profound wisdom, integrity, and honesty within this community could be brought to bear on so many other problems. It seems to me that a "University of Ethics, Responsibility, Community, and Love" could be built in the Castro. Students there could learn from masters.

Even I, stubborn creature that I am, have learned a few of these spiritual lessons. I, too, have discovered unexpected sources of hope and learned anew the value of other sources of hope that have been with me throughout my life.

For one thing, I have seen a deepening of my spiritual understandings about life, suffering, and death. I don't pretend to have the words for those understandings yet, but I am buoyed by them. In yielding to the knowledge that my life and my sense of myself have changed, I am released a bit from the need to protect myself from further change. As I accept the possibility of change in my life, and even death, I lose the illusion that I am a permanent facility in this world. I find freedom in that as well as fear and wonderment.

I am convinced that we must feel something to know it is real. I have felt change deeply in my bones as well as in my soul; that experiential knowledge is often steadying and gives me hope.

I draw still more hope from an image that keeps coming to me, one which has sustained me through the years. Whenever I feel shaky about my future, our collective future, or that of the earth, I think of the children I have seen going off to school all over the world. In Korea, India, South Africa, Vietnam, and the United States I see children with their shirts tucked in, the holes in the knees of their pants mended, their books in some kind of a bag, their hair combed. Someone has dressed these children as well as they can afford, has braided or combed their hair, has helped prepare them for the day. Someone has set learning as a priority over other economic uses of this child. From this I get the sense that the world is being passed on with some kind of care and love.

And it's love, most of all, which keeps my hope alive. Most of my life I have been well loved; this year has been no exception. As in most years there have been some less than wonderful parts of the loving—by me as well as toward me. But on the whole I have been awarely cared for by my friends, by those close enough to be called family, and by my family. They have allowed me to love them as much as they are able. And I have allowed them to love me to the best of my capacity.

We are growing into knowing how to love in these times. The mistakes are natural and are by far preferable to not loving at all. The love I see in the world and in myself is a great source of hope for me.

Finally, my hope is in today—one day at a time. I have no idea what tomorrow will bring, but I have a sense that I will find within myself and my social and natural context the resources to get through it. Because I have changed this year, I am confident I can change tomorrow. If I knew now what tomorrow would hold, I probably would not choose it. But I know I will find my way through it and probably be just about as happy as I am today. It is my dreams that give life meaning, not my nightmares.

It is my experience with myself that my happiness is not so much circumstance-determined as related to my inner resources. I have found the resources to pass through this year with happiness often enough at my side so that I have not forgotten her face. This makes me believe that she is a friend for life. And if my suffering becomes so intense that I lose her for awhile, I pray I will see her in the face of my friends, the mountains, trees, and rivers so that I know she is out there somewhere.

Collected Writings on AIDS

On Secrets

W hen I first found out I was HIV+ I thought I could never tell anyone, I was so afraid. I've heard that HIV-infected women on the average only tell two people about their situation. I had somehow picked up that this virus was not only a horrible thing to have, but a person would be rejected and ostracized by others if the condition became known; therefore it was best to keep quiet. Over the months I have slowly found my way to understanding where this fear came from in myself, and I have walked into a new understanding of the role of secrecy in life. As any HIV+ person will tell you, we have to deal with very intimate issues involving our health and sex lives; and we experience corresponding changes in our "extimate" lives as the society around us evidences such fear about this virus.

Given the level of hysteria in America at this time, it is realistic to expect that some people will be hostile and rejecting if they find out about one's HIV status. I have met many people now who have been asked to leave jobs, 12-step programs, intimate relationships, apartments, even doctor/patient relationships when it became known that they were "carriers"—a word which I have really come to hate.

In putting my name on this book I have realized that my situation is unique. I am secure in my home. I have my life's work but no job as such. As time has gone on, my relationship with my doctor has convinced me that she will stand by me through this. In general, my experience is that when people realize I am HIV+, some move closer while other dear and old friends fade into the fabric of the past. On some occasions I have run into such fear and blind prejudice that I have been hesitant to write about these experiences. I had a house guest from Canada who, upon discovering I was HIV+, left the house rather than get or trust any information about his safety. One

125

man I have known for ten years refused to allow his children to be close to me.

With each close friend, the scenario in the months after finding out I was positive went something like this:

"Hi, how are you doing?" they would say.

"Fine, how about you?" I would say rather automatically. After all, they hadn't really asked how I was; it's a formality. We would talk for awhile. Internally I would be feeling more and more uncomfortable. "This person doesn't even know what I am going through—that I live in a land they have not known me to be in. I am sitting here looking like a normal person, yet I have a deep pain inside or me—and they don't even know. I look just as I always have looked to them. Am I doing a good job of covering up what I am really feeling and thinking? They can't tell. I don't want them to know. But then it would be a relief to share this with somebody. It feels lonely in here right now, sitting alone with these questions and fears. How would they feel if they knew I had something going on inside of me right now that I feel uncomfortable sharing with them? They would think I didn't trust them. Well, I don't! What would they do if they knew? Would they still be my friend? Would they be willing and able to share some of the load I am carrying? No, probably not. They would like me to be the reliable Fran Peavey they have always known. Besides, right now we are busy doing whatever we are doing. Best not to rock the boat. And anyway what does this person know about HIV? Nothing except what they read in the papers. Would they be my friend if they knew I was hiding from them the most important thing that is happening in my life right now? Will they feel I did not have confidence in them if they find out in a few months or years that I knew about being HIV+ all this time? Will they worry if I share this apple? If I don't tell them, it doesn't leave them in charge of their lives or let them make decisions of how much risk they want to take. Still I know what the risks are, and maybe I can be careful for us both. But they might make a different decision about sharing this apple. And besides, does anybody know about the risks for sure? I had better not take a bite—not because I think it would be dangerous to them, but because I don't want to worry them—even though they don't know about it all at this point. Maybe I should just tell her/him...I hate this feeling of hiding, of dishonesty and un-connection in the presence of another. I feel so far away. Is there a way I can get closer—without telling about my life and what HIV is putting me through? Probably not...."

In the early group of four which I convened at church, one woman—Karen—seemed particularly insightful on issues of "disclosure" (as they say in HIV-ese). So I named her my "Openness Consultant." Each time I was confronted with a situation where I felt my relationship was being compromised by holding this secret, I would call her. She would help me explore what it would mean to tell the person, what it would mean not to tell, and how I felt about both options.

The general policy I have come to about "disclosure" for myself is that I tell people when I feel "my situation" is interfering with our relationship, or if at the moment I am thinking about it in a way that prevents me from being fully with the other person. I look at it like this: If I am creating or carrying a stone which will sit between us and interfere with our relating to each other in the deepest and most human way possible in any given moment, my task is to decide whether I need that stone for my own protection or whether I can remove it, thus moving a little more truth into our relationship. Then we will have a more open channel to be with each other. I don't tell people if I think "it would interest them" or if just now I want to ignore this part of my life and live a "normal life."

There are secrets I have not included in this journal. Things happened pretty quickly there for a while. I don't seem to have written about the conversation I had with a friend about euthanasia, for instance. This conversation allowed me to rest knowing that I would have help and companionship should I decide I needed to end my life. My friend agreed to procure a pill which would be an adequate and painless poison, and to help me think through the decision to take it. Now I don't really think about the issue since I believe it is resolved. It was a calm conversation about how people with AIDS die (usually it seems to be a long and slow death) and how my economic and relationship base would only allow for a limited time of downhill spiral. When I feel that base stretched too far, I plan to stop.

I have not told you of the hateful thoughts I have occasionally about individuals. With this "new weapon"—my own blood—I do sometimes think "I should just go and bleed on them." It seems kind of funny now, but I do think those things from time to time when someone cuts in front of me on the freeway or hurts me. I often experience free-floating anger about carrying this virus, and I would be less than honest if I did not acknowledge that anger. It hurts me that I am surrounded by people standing on a safe shore that I do not know how to reach.

But there is a more disturbing secretiveness for me about this HIV business. It involves my relationship to the institutions upon which I must rely to stay healthy and sane. From my first visit to Lisa, my HIV medical consultant, I have used a false name in all registrations and conversations. I have this foreboding feeling (is it paranoia or not—I cannot tell) that having my name on record as being HIV+ could be to my disadvantage someday.

So how does this false identity affect my life? On my answering machine now I say "This is Fran Peavey. —— and I are out; leave a message," since medical institutions call leaving messages giving me information and reminding me about appointments. Friends ask who "she" is, assuming I have a new roommate or lover. Each time I go to an appointment I have a new small dread that I will forget "my name" or be faced with someone who recognizes me. But on a deeper level, I believe that using this false name creates a lack of harmony in myself which I do not feel promotes my wellness. I do not feel myself to be a whole person connected with my history, present in my own skin, when I go to deal with this difficult situation. I sense my integrity is being compromised.

I continue to deliberate about the exposure issues involved in the Gann initiative as I write this book, which surely will be more exposing than the registering required in the proposed law. There is a world of difference between the state wanting information for its own purposes of controlling people and a book communicating a whole story and point of view. How will you, dear reader, feel about me now? If you come to a comedy performance will you see me and think, "There is a sick person"? I hope not because I am not sick. Will you think you are inadequate to the task of talking with me because you do not know how to face your own fear of the epidemic? Will I become more of a symbol of this epidemic than a real person? When I make a mistake will you think, "She's slipping. Probably dementia is setting in"? I hope not, because I have always made my share of mistakes.

I intend to continue to take risks and do things I don't know how to do yet. Risk-taking often involves making some mistakes in the learning process. I can't stop learning new things or taking risks because of my own fear that you (or I) will attribute these mistakes to a worsening of the illness. When I mess up, will you let me know and share your anger with me just as you always have, or now that you think I might die someday, will you just let it go? And will you be afraid to get close to me or other HIV+ people because you fear "getting the virus" or because you are apprehensive that we will die and leave you? The real tragedy is that fear would keep us from being friends and opening to each other in any way that makes sense to us.

Or will you become an intimacy voyeur, thrusting yourself into a close space with me to get some hit of tragedy and depth which you lack in your own life? And will you then walk away glad that you can escape my day-to-day reality?

Even at this moment as I write this, a woman stops by to see an apartment in the house I live in. She says she recognizes me. We have met getting our hair cut. She says, "Now that I'm out of school I must read your book. Are your writing any more?"

"Yes, in fact I am finishing one in there right now," I reply, motioning toward the office in my house as I walk in the garden.

"Oh, what is it about?"

"Well, it will be called *A Shallow Pool of Time* (I am buying time here trying to think how to say what this book is about) and it is about what is happening in our time, you know, social hysteria, waiting, my work, and there is some historical stuff on AIDS." (Have I hidden the AIDS stuff enough in the brush so she doesn't think I have any personal knowledge about the world of AIDS?)

Hiding is hard on a person. And it's an even harder habit to break.

Face of AIDS

The Face of AIDS

I see the face of AIDS
  in my world on every continent
    in my country in every state
      in my city in each neighborhood.

I see the face of AIDS
  It is a face contorted in fear
    a deep fear
      of blood
        of sex
          of death
            of homosexuals
              fear of Africans and Haitians
                fear of people different from the self.

              Plague in our times
              In our family
                Can you believe it?

Terror in newspaper headlines
    national and municipal budgets stretched
    insurance companies unable to cope with the bills
    johns unwilling to use condoms for their illicit pleasure
    parents unable to control their children's sexual explorations
  Ignorance and fear mixed as thick as peanut butter.

I see the face of AIDS,
    it is a face thin, old, worn before its time
      eyes receding in their sockets
        staring beyond the thin veil of present reality
      seeing a life beyond and unsure of the route.

I see the face of AIDS
    a baby born of a virus-infested woman,
      a baby needing love
        yet abandoned by a mother too ill to care.
    But of course mothers are never too ill to really care
      about losing life
        their babies'
        or their own.
I see the face of AIDS in the quiet saint of our times
    who steps forward to care for this babe,
      for the mother,
      for all infected
        for as long as they shall live.

I see the face of AIDS
    in my neighbor who comes home from the hospital
      in an ambulance
    to the arms of his lover who carries him into the house
      like a bride
    They live out their lives in quiet retreat together
      sleeping in the same bed
      each terrified of going on alone.

I see the face of AIDS
    in the outraged crowd gathering to protest
      too high a price
      being charged for an elixir which offers hope to the
        hopeless.

I see the face of AIDS everywhere now on the streets of my world
    because I see it in myself
      one of the worried well.

October 12, 1988

Dear Tourist

Dear Tourist,

Welcome to San Francisco. Those of us who live here are happy to share our beautiful city with you. We have written this guide so that you can "share the San Francisco experience" as we approach the last decade of the twentieth century.

There are really many San Franciscos, as we live in neighborhoods and identify ourselves in that way. The Mission District, Noe Valley, the Sunset, the Castro, the Richmond, Chinatown—the list goes on. Recently a particular San Francisco experience cuts across all neighborhoods, all classes, and across all racial and ethnic lines. It is almost an underground phenomenon, and is largely invisible to the casual observer—whether they live here and simply are uninvolved, or are visitors who cannot see the depth of life being lived behind the bay windows of this City by the Bay. It has become one of the dominant San Francisco experiences. It is the experience of living with an epidemic—AIDS.

The word "epidemic" is sometimes used so casually these days that you may not realize what it means in this place. According to Mayor Art Agnos, we have lost *twice as many* of our citizens—men and women too—in this decade to AIDS than our city lost in World War I and II, the Korean war, and the Vietnamese war combined! Because AIDS so profoundly touches each of us whether we are personally HIV+ or not, it is fair to say that our city has AIDS. What does this mean in the lives of the people you see on our streets, the people who serve you in restaurants and shops?

It means that most of us are grieving in one way or another. We have recently lost someone we cared about. And probably there have been many more funerals in our recent past. We have lost some of our most creative, energetic, and artistic friends. And we miss them, individually and collectively.

It also means that probably each institution and many people you meet who live here spend some of their resources, some of their time, and money, helping people with AIDS (PWAs). Restaurants probably assist with the food program if they are community minded. Many stores will display a sign as you walk in giving PWAs a 10 to 15 percent discount on purchases. Many of the people you meet spend 5 to 10 hours (and some lots more than that) volunteering in organizations that provide a vast array of services (vacuuming, walking PWA's dogs, cooking, writing wills, counseling and offering emotional support, driving people to the hospital, and a myriad of other things) for those people who no longer have the energy to do these essential tasks for themselves.

But in a larger sense, as you walk on our streets you encounter people grappling very deeply with feelings of helplessness at not being able to stop all the dying in this place. For most of us this is an intensely private time. We are sometimes afraid that people will reject us if they know our relation to AIDS. We fear that people not directly impacted by the virus really don't care about our losses here. You are among people who are dying, who love people who are dying, and yet all of these people are living—and most of them feel their life to be very much with them. We are a city *living* with AIDS.

While you are with us don't worry. You can't get this virus from walking around on our streets. We invite you to come to Castro Street, in the neighborhood most severely impacted, and walk with us. Come to our restaurants and shops, our churches, our theater. Possibly you will feel the intense connectedness we have as we work together to live, to help each other, and to stop this wild fire threatening us all. As you walk on Castro you can think to yourself that about every third person you meet probably has the AIDS virus roaming around inside. You can't get this virus from breathing the air we breathe. It is spread via blood and sexual contact. You can't get it from food prepared by HIV+ hands (even if the cook accidentally cut himself, the virus can't enter your system through the digestive tract). You can't get it from our toilet seats or from the very few mosquitoes we have.

Of course, we would strongly encourage you to use safe sex in this city, whether you love a man or a woman. You should do that everywhere in the world now in new relationships until you can be sure of the status of your partner. You are among a people who have learned to make enormous changes in their lives in order to be socially responsible people. The spread of AIDS in the Gay community has been significantly slowed by a determined effort on the part of the community. We have a certain sense of pride that we have been able to change aspects of our life which are important to us and still find great joy in our lives.

So while you are here with us, enter into our special sense of time. We are here, now—and may not be tomorrow. Isn't that really always true? Here you have the opportunity to be with people who know that special, almost sacred, time between the awareness that death is approaching and their actual dying. Let us share with you our dignity in the face of prejudice and fear, and the powerful sense of community which has developed for us in the turbulence of this epidemic. Let us tell you how it feels to have so many names in our address book crossed out recently and to miss these people so intensely that we often feel we have lost the ability to cry any more. Many of us have been to more funerals in our lifetime than our grandparents. Sometimes it seems there is so much grieving to do that it is hard to do any. There is so much loving to be done, that it's a struggle to stop to take care of mundane things. We have so much living to do that we are very busy enjoying life now. Please join with us. This is the San Francisco experience in the 1980s.

"An audit by the National Gay and Lesbian Task Force in Washington, D.C., shows reports of crimes (against gays) and harassment have more than tripled in three years, from 2,042 cases in 1985 to 7,008 cases last year"..."AIDS is responsible for the upsurge in gay bashing, gay activists say" ... "A meeting with conservative Rep. Bob Dornan, R-Buena Park, deteriorated into a shouting match, with the Republican congressman's wife, Sallie, yelling, "Shut up, fag" to a gay activist. Later, she emotionally apologized and said the remark came out of anger over the fact that one of her four brothers was dying of AIDS. Bob Dornan, who said he didn't know about his brother-in-law's illness, still holds an anti-gay stance."
—*San Francisco Examiner*, October 9, 1988

If we pay attention, we can see the warning signs: the increase in gay-bashing, the outbursts of political leaders, the ballot initiatives targeting people with AIDS. In 1987 the Ku Klux Klan called for homosexual men to be interned in camps to stop AIDS. But it is not just the lunatic fringe that has taken up the cause of persecuting gays and other people in AIDS target groups. One of the reasons Proposition 102 was so frightening was that it was sponsored not by someone like Lyndon LaRouche, but by leaders in California's Republican party.

These are the warning signs of social hysteria. For much of my life I have been trying to understand the phenomenon of social hysteria: what happens when a society, under stress, loses its balance. Social hysteria is when people lose it in a collective way and do things that are against their true nature. I trace my interest in social hysteria back to my childhood, when I frequently accompanied my father on his trips around Idaho's Magic Valley. He supervised farms for a Dutch land company, and we would drive around from farm to farm, talking together, eating potatoes freshly dug from the ground—raw, sliced with Dad's pocket knife and salted from a shaker he kept in the glove compartment for just such moments. Often he would get sad as we passed a group of low-lying army barracks just outside Paul, Idaho. He explained to me that these were the prisons, politely called internment camps, where American citizens of Japanese descent had been held during World War II.

My father would invariably say something like, "When bad times come, people become frightened and do things they would never do in ordinary circumstances. Governments even do things against their own laws. In bad times, some people become more generous, think more about other people's needs, and become better people. Others become mean, selfish, greedy, and think only of themselves."

I am at the older edge of the group that is loosely called "the Baby Boomers." (We have also been called the "Hippies," the "Me Generation," and the "Yuppies.") Those of us born after World War II have moved through each phase of life leaving our mark, partly because of our large numbers and partly because we carry in our collective consciousness certain powerful historical events. Many of these events relate directly to the question of social hysteria.

My generation grew up in the shadow of the Holocaust, asking itself why Nazism arose in Germany. Could such a thing happen here? The social hysteria of that time took root in conditions of economic depression, and was exploited by people with a sick political and social agenda. The German people were told by their leaders that certain groups—the Jews, the leftists, the homosexuals—were the cause of the bad economic times.

Another historical reference point for my generation is the McCarthy period. As I was studying the Bill of Rights with its promises of free speech and freedom of assembly, I remember my parents being glued to the radio listening to hearings in Washington. These hearings did not square at all with what I was learning in school. Now it is the consensus that those were dark times for my country.

My generation's relationship to social hysteria is also shaped by our experience with polio. Growing up, we survived by not swimming in pools after a certain month, not drinking from fountains, and by engaging in various other practices thought to keep us safe. But I—and I suspect most people now over 40—lost classmates to this epidemic. Pictures of iron lungs, poster boys with braces on their legs and crutches, were burned into our minds. My cousin Alex died of polio, and I remember the fear that sat at our dining room table that week. But most of us survived the polio epidemic. When we reached adulthood, in addition to being able to drink beer, we could eat one pink sugar cube with a vaccine inside it and be safe for the rest of our lives—or so they said at the time. For twenty years or so we had the illusion of invulnerability from plague. What a time it was! We took that freedom and ran with it. Having had that freedom makes it all the harder to break through our denial and face a new epidemic and the changes in our sex lives that are now necessary.

Since social hysteria often occurs against a backdrop of economic hard times, it is significant that my generation has had little experience with such hardship. The fifties and sixties were, for the most part, boom times. We came of age expecting it all—cars, houses, dishwashers, and so on. But as a professor at San Francisco State University in the early 1970s, I led a workshop with teachers and administrators that raised troubling questions about the social fear that would be stirred by economic constriction.

In the workshop, we were studying different scenarios for the future; at one point a heated argument erupted which nearly ended in a physical fight between two groups. One group presented a scenario of unlimited growth, a future which dramatically conflicted with the scenario of limited resources presented by the other group. As I watched them shout at each other and saw the rage build in my classroom, I experienced a chain of thoughts something like this: "These people are not going joyfully into the future, willing to limit their consumption. We are deeply addicted to our lifestyle, and to the stuff in our lives. Having to consume less will deeply disturb our social fabric. People in the Third World are going to see our standard of living on television and rightfully demand more for their labor, and a greater share of the resources taken from their countries. This combined with the loss of a clean and safe environment due to pollution caused by our industries and lifestyle...*Oh dear.*"

I felt as though I were seeing two airplanes headed toward each other on a collision course. It did not seem that the American people—my people—were going to diminish their expectations easily. I sensed that it was going to be a very painful—a pathologically painful—transition. Fortunately, dinnertime came and the fight that was building was broken up for a while. When we reassembled, we all talked about how frightening this rage had been for us. I learned a lot that night.

A condition such as AIDS, which is difficult to understand and which involves factors perceived as beyond control, laden with symbolic overload, inherently carries a high potential for social hysteria. But what is most dangerous is that in our country the epidemic affects primarily those who have already been defined by the dominant culture as the "other." In her book *Blaming Others*, Renée Sabatier writes:

> "Seven years into the AIDS epidemic in the United States, it is becoming clear that what was originally perceived as a disease of white middle-class homosexuals has also been the unnoticed tragedy of the minorities, the disadvantaged, and the disenfranchised. Among white adults in the United States, the incidence of AIDS cases is 189 per million population; for blacks it

is 578 per million; and for Hispanics it is 564 per million...These figures mean that a black or Hispanic person in the United States is 3 times more likely to have AIDS than a white."

AIDS disproportionately affects people from groups made marginal by society, groups that lack political power. How easy it is to blame the epidemic on its victims—the impoverished drug users, the homosexuals, the immigrants from the Caribbean and Africa. Most Americans have lots of psychological distance from these people. According to Susan Sontag in the *New York Review of Books*, plagues through the ages have been thought to have come from somewhere else.

Once the target groups are defined, it is easy to scapegoat them. Scapegoating allows the social system to assign blame for a bad situation, to focus its energy on attacking the targeted group rather than on attending to the sources of the problems. If the increased gay bashing and the California ballot initiatives are any indication, the scapegoating and stigmatizing have already begun.

I received seven harassing telephone calls, all anonymous, after an article appeared in the newspaper about the reasons I was critical of the Gann initiative. Of course I dismiss these callers as people sick with fear and ignorance; but they are still forces in my world, and their fear impacts me very directly. Their hysteria is an illness that can be transmitted over the phone, on the airwaves, in the voting booth.

There are more subtle indications of the societal shift, as well. Recently I saw a newspaper headline—"Man With AIDS in Holdup." This headline may not seem ludicrous until one considers the opposite: "Man Without AIDS in Holdup." Just because a person specializing in holdups gets AIDS does not mean he will get a new line of work. Headlines like these can serve to deepen prejudice and social hysteria.

No period of social hysteria is quite like any other. I do not, for example, foresee HIV+ people being taken to ovens. But in times of social hysteria there seem to be certain predictable manifestations of the terror just below the surface:

- an increase in random street violence;
- yellow journalism, which fans the hysteria;
- political opportunism;
- a sense of urgency that we simply do not "have the time" to arrive at a national (or group) consensus—that decisions must be made quickly;
- social and/or legal constraints on dissent;

- the rise of cults with leaders who ask people to believe and act in accord with group norms rather than trusting their own intelligence; and
- controlling legislation.

We must face the possibility that a society in the early stages of social hysteria can resist the attack only so long. Like a virus hidden in a computer program and timed to go off at a specific moment, in any given society there are viruses in the collective psyche which can go off and threaten the health of the body politic. Then the system breaks down and becomes vulnerable to opportunistic infections.

If health insurance companies flounder, if municipal governments find themselves impossibly stretched to meet hospital bills for this epidemic, then the social hysteria we see beginning now may reach its awful potential. Populations identified with AIDS may be seen as needing to be controlled; society may decide to take them, against their will, into prisons—even if these prisons are called relocation centers or "hospitals."

In 1982 I attended a conference on holocaust and genocide, held in Tel Aviv. Most of the participants were Jewish survivors of Nazi concentration camps; there were also presentations made by Armenians and Tibetans. At the conference I learned an important lesson: creating laws to protect people who are being targeted in periods of social hysteria does not prevent governments and individuals from doing horrible and illegal things. So although it is important to pass legislation protecting the rights of HIV+ people, the legislation by itself is not enough.

The most powerful antidote to social hysteria is community: people acting together, with all our strengths and vulnerability, sharing resources both human and material. Human beings are the agar plate on which the bacteria of social hysteria grows—or fails to grow. Each of us is a part of our social context; each of us helps to create the environment in which historical developments occur.

When my father and I drove past the site of the Japanese-American internment camps, he regularly gave me this advice: "Always live so that you can be generous in bad times; you will have more fun with your friends and will feel better about yourself when the bad times end. And bad times always do end. When good times return, people remember the people who were greedy; they remember their choices and they don't feel good about how they acted."

In the paragraphs that follow, I offer some specific suggestions for minimizing social hysteria. These ideas are drawn from my years of working as a nonviolent activist as well as a consultant on social change.

Keep channels of good information open. To fight the rumors and misinformation which fuel social hysteria, we need reliable sources of information that are easily accessible. Telephone hotlines, newsletters, speakers who criss-cross the nation sharing new ideas and perspectives, computer conferences on AIDS, and educational organizations are all vital. When you hear "facts" about AIDS which you are skeptical of, call the AIDS hotline, 800-342-AIDS. They have current information, and can answer questions and refer you to local resources.

Humanize the issue. Avoid talking about AIDS only in abstract terms. In conversations, mention your personal connection with the epidemic: for example, "My brother-in-law had AIDS." Abstract conversations take the humanity out of the issue and feed hysteria. People who carry the virus should consider "coming out" to all those they can trust not to harm them. This is of strategic value: people need to see the face of AIDS, to put their fear into perspective, to remember that there are real human beings being affected. Empathy is one of the most powerful antidotes to social hysteria.

When discussing AIDS, concentrate on "I" statements. In conversations, when you hear people talk about "what those people are doing," speak in the first person: "I am wondering what I can do to teach my children about safe sex." Stay with yourself and your relationship to the problem; don't project fear onto others.

Focus on risky behaviors rather than people in "high risk groups." Anyone in any social or racial group can get AIDS if they engage in certain practices. Challenge all socially irresponsible practices which can spread the virus. Safe sex and clean needles are imperative.

Commit yourself to being a nonviolent ally of AIDS people. Strong nonviolent actions are a key to stopping social hysteria. Do something positive about the situation on a regular basis so that you continue to feel connected and active. If you are HIV+, those panic attacks that we are so familiar with need to be talked about, and actions found to keep them under control. I felt much less fearful about the Gann ballot initiative when I started working against it.

Do not settle for information given to you by the media about this epidemic. Volunteer to help people with AIDS or the organizations which serve them, so you can get information firsthand. Hundreds of organizations are working on this epidemic, and they need all kinds of skills, from clerical and medical support to housecleaning and dog walking.

Wake yourself up while watching images of AIDS on television.
Taking in frightening information on TV can be an isolating and
passive experience. The contrast of one's comfortable home and life
with that of the people with AIDS shown on television sets up a
dissonance which feeds hysteria. Think about the images of AIDS
you carry in your mind: men with sunken eyes on hospital beds,
barely able to raise their heads. This looks mysterious and frightening to most people. Think how these images affect your perceptions
of AIDS. Television rarely shows the women and children, or the
active PWAs exercising at the gym, working at their jobs, eating in
a restaurant. I have met PWAs who are: a woman professor in a
major medical school, collections agents, a comptroller, mothers,
grandmothers, children, a millionaire, a computer consultant, a
janitor, a male nurse, a products delivery person, salesmen, an
actress, and a woman farmer.

**Be gentle with yourself as you take in new information, grow, and
change.** In an area where fear is present, people can become so afraid
of having been "wrong" yesterday that they cut themselves off from
the chance of being more "right" tomorrow. We are just beginning
to learn how to live with this disease, and none of us has it completely
figured out yet. Practice patience with yourself as well as with
others.

**Actively support public officials or institutions taking respon-
sible positions on AIDS.** They will be enduring criticism and need
to know that there is support out there for them. Write them, call
their offices, promote their products, and let them know that you are
supporting them because of their position on AIDS.

**Support policies which give people with AIDS dignity, security,
protection, and control of their lives.** Welcome PWAs in your
family gatherings, groups, churches and work places. Don't make
someone your "pet PWA," but find concrete ways to express your
acceptance. Learn to value their contribution. They are looking at the
world through a set of lenses that give them a particular kind of
wisdom. To the degree that most PWAs feel a part of the social fabric,
they will find creative ways of being responsible.

Some aspects of my experience with this plague have helped
restore my confidence in humanity. I have seen the words of my
father confirmed in the bad times of my generation, as some individuals reach past their fear and small-mindedness to find a remarkable nobility and generosity of spirit. Instead of touching the pain of

AIDS with fear, people have found ways to touch it with love. The deep sense of community I have seen rising from this terror is unmatched in my experience.

Shortly after I got my test results, I discovered that, outside of hospitals, there were no homes for women with AIDS to spend their last days. AIDS hospices existed for men, but not for women. I called together a few friends and we began working to raise money for residential services for women. The enthusiasm and dedication of our group has astonished me.

The volunteer infrastructure in San Francisco is incredible. People give massages to AIDS patients, clean their houses, carry responsibility for emotional support, even share their financial resources. Some PWAs who can no longer tolerate certain medications continue to get these expensive pills with their insurance payments and turn them over to an underground distribution network, which gets the pills to others who cannot afford them. In one company, workers pooled their vacation time and gave it to an AIDS patient so that he would not lose his job for being sick so long.

There is something very potent about focused collective action. It helps people mend their fear and stay connected with their compassion. It reestablishes people's confidence that they can be counted on to alleviate suffering. And a self-confident people is a revolutionary people—willing and able to make change.

In the long run, wounds heal, and sanity returns to systems. This virus may be the challenge to our alienation that allows us to learn, at last, just how dependent we are on one another. I do believe that we human beings are really a decent and good bunch, and that we can be brought to a collective mindfulness of our delicate and fragile situation.

On Waiting

There is an old myth from India which speaks very much to our condition today. It is about the huma bird, a magical creature that lives in the remotest reaches of the stratosphere and which, from birth to death, never touches ground or tree. It eats, sleeps, hunts, and mates in flight. From the loftiest heights the mother lays her egg in the air. The egg starts falling. Any observers in that mythical realm would certainly shudder in fear to see that helpless newborn plummeting toward certain death. The egg plunges faster and faster toward the earth; but as it falls, the embryo inside is rapidly taking form, rapidly growing; its little body is developing, its feet, head and wings are taking form. As its beak becomes hard, it starts to peck away at the inside of the shell. Suddenly the shell bursts open and the baby chick emerges into the world to find itself hurtling like a meteor towards disaster. But as the ground looms ever larger and closer in its sight, the newborn feels its little wings unfolding, and its feathers grow and dry out. Just in the split second before it crashes to the ground—to instant annihilation—it flaps its tiny new wings and flies up, up, up into the sky to join its mother in the highest heavens, far above the clouds.

Many of us feel like the huma bird these days. How are we going to get out of the egg of our despair and spiritual immaturity? For some of us our beaks are not hardened. Others of us wonder if our wings will dry quickly enough to fly us back to safety—together and individually. We are right in the middle of that period when we can see that the old is dead, and yet we don't quite know what the new is that is trying to be born. We yearn to see from inside the egg the bird that we will be, to know whether we will mature and fly or be dashed to the ground.

Some friends have suggested that I keep this journal going until I die—then it would make a "great book." But I didn't want to wait that long to publish this material. You see, I plan to live for quite a while.

As I prepare this book for publication, I find it illuminating to read back on the journal entries from five years ago and to reflect on the changes I have seen in our society, in my friendship network, and of

145

course in myself regarding this epidemic. I have experienced the testing and tearing at the fabric of community caused by the AIDS epidemic. I have seen that tearing from both sides—as a person watching the epidemic from the sidelines, and then as a person caught up in the epidemic. Rereading the early journal entries has given me a new appreciation of the position of the bystander, but by the end of this writing I have come to realize that none of us is really a bystander. We all participate in this epidemic, whatever our perspective.

AIDS has offered me, and others in our early or middle years, the challenge to live more consciously. I can't say that the grass has been greener or the sun warmer since I became aware of this virus' presence inside me. I cannot say that it has enriched my human relationships or made me more trusting, though I have become more discerning about people's ability to deal with fear. Friends have told me that I am a sweeter and more open person lately. I am amazed at these reports and wonder how these friends could have missed my sweetness before.

My test results thrust me into the gay and lesbian community in a way that I could not have anticipated. I have come to respect and love the gay community in San Francisco, and to admire the humanity with which they—we—are facing this plague.

This book ends with more questions and greater uncertainty than it began with. And the uncertainty is formidable. A growing number of people are HIV+. Many others are suffering from various mysterious ailments, including candida, chronic fatigue immune dysfunctional syndrome (sometimes know as Epstein-Barr virus), and all kinds of allergies and environmental illnesses. Is the suffering in the world increasing, am I simply growing older, or is something happening to our species? I can't help speculating that we human beings have created a biosphere which we can no longer tolerate. The non-human species are not the only ones under threat from our modern way of life. It is us, too.

I love to walk among great, old trees. Last summer a friend took me to a maple forest in Vermont. As we walked my friend told me that a healthy maple tree has a full leaf pattern in its outer perimeter, so its outline creates a solid, rather smooth line. You don't see spaces between the branches. From the jagged line of foliage on nearly all of the trees, it was easy to see that this forest was gravely ill. Like other forests in Canada and the northeastern United States, it has been poisoned by acid rain.

I hear that three quarters of the people in my spiritual community in San Francisco have the AIDS virus in their blood. On Sundays when I stand to sing, I look around and sense that I am standing in a dying forest. I miss trees from month to month. Friends are falling all around me.

We live in a world that is too polluted. There is not enough of an ozone layer left to protect us. Too much radioactivity has been released. New viruses mutate, or are man-made; new conditions threaten our species.

It seems that we do not yet know how to mourn and let go when a whole way of life begins to die. Even when we can see that death, can know it from inside, it is difficult to believe that a new way of life must and will emerge. In these last years of the twentieth century, our old way of life has already begun its terminal decline, and yet we do not see a new birth arising.

We do not know how to mourn this death. So automatically, and in something of a frenzy, we cling to that which is mostly dead. It is our clinging that most surely will kill us, or at least speed the downward spiral.

Maybe we people who carry the AIDS virus are the canaries in the mine. Maybe we can whistle such a true and sweet song that our species will see that we must get out of the mine; we must change our addiction to consumption, pollution and mindlessness.

I, and thousands like me with viruses in our bodies, are waiting. This is not a passive waiting: we are not resigned to death. In many ways we are busy doing whatever we can to increase our chances of "beating this thing," as Dennis put it. But there is a lot of waiting, too.

When I visited South Africa in 1986 I saw an entire society that was, in a sense, waiting. The black South Africans I spoke with showed a curious mixture of hope and hopelessness. They wait for the spark that will ignite a new level of struggle and offer a new possibility of change in the social contract between peoples. The white South Africans wait for that, too—sensing, perhaps dreading, the deep suffering and change that is in store for them when the inevitable spark comes. But they find hope within hopelessness as they look north at Zimbabwe where whites and blacks have passed through a revolution and now live in a new social arrangement where both racial groups participate in decisions in a way that is new for them.

The South Africans' way of waiting—of carrying on with faith and hope in the face of individually hopeless situations—was a perspective I personally had only dimly understood; became clearer to me this summer as I wrestled with the waiting that lay before me, as I wondered what this AIDS virus was doing in my body. Contemplating my own future and our collective future—both very much in doubt—I asked myself, "How can I learn to wait, to sit with the devastating information which I now know?"

When I give talks or do comedy shows, people often approach me afterward to ask me about the future. They take me to a corner of the room and quietly say, "I hear that the environment is so destroyed that it cannot be reversed, that the end has already begun. Is that true?" They think somehow a comedian will know! Turning to comedians with questions like that is like putting clowns at the health centers to tell people whether they are HIV+. (Maybe that's not a bad idea!) What can I tell these people? I have read about studies by the Worldwatch Institute and by the United Nations which indicate that some parts of our ecosystems and some species have been irreversibly destroyed. But who can know the extent of the damage? Our physical world is so complex and interconnected that the ramifications of any deterioration are significant and, I suspect, more extensive than most of us can comprehend.

And so we wait. Our waiting is directed toward a questionable future, one that seems to be closing in on the present and making it untenable. We are waiting for something we really don't want. We do everything we can to postpone the expected future. A friend of mine told me that before he knew he was HIV+ he jogged furiously every day, hoping that he could "outrun" the virus. As a species, we try to clean up toxic waste dumps and stop the clear cutting of the forests. We make every effort to preserve our health and our planet, but we also must wait, knowing the virus is already in the system, not yet knowing whether it is terminal or not. All actions may increase the odds that the ecosystem will not collapse completely before key changes can be brought into place.

Still, this waiting can feel like a passive activity. It produces in us feelings of powerlessness and vulnerability—infantile feelings—and we hate that. We rage against our powerlessness, our vulnerability, our having to wait. It is from this rage that measures like the Gann public health initiative arise. It is this rage that fuels the discussion of violent strategies in the AIDS community. In both instances, the rage is born of despair and a weariness of waiting while suffering continues.

In our times there is a prevalent sense of "resignation", as Robert Lifton calls it. I occasionally taste the pungent flavor of that resignation myself. I have been looking at this resignation, within me, exploring it, trying to find out how to work with that resignation in order to allow my beak to harden so I can peck my way out of my egg and grow up and fly. It is a very tough task. In the early days of working against nuclear war and environmental destruction, I decided to ask myself every day the strategic question, "What can I do to help the world survive?" Since then I have made it my practice to get up usually between four and five in the morning, sitting for an hour with that question, as well as practicing loving people I am separated from.

I thought in 1979 that I might have to ask this question for many years without receiving any ideas from that life force inside and outside me. But I was willing to give the life force an opportunity to create answers and to develop my will by first walking answerless into the void of my morning sitting. I was prepared to do that for ten years without an answer. I said to myself that if at the end of that time no answer had come, I would re-evaluate. This is the tenth year of that practice. Fortunately some answers have arrived including comedy and other projects that I work on today. To be willing to ask strategic questions to which there are no known answers, and to wait—those are among the most difficult and heroic tasks we can do now. To continue to ask and consult that universal life force to direct us is, I believe, one of the most valuable beak-hardening and spiritually-maturing tasks we can do in our time.

We also must be willing to do whatever the life-force-from-within suggests. Often only a small thing comes clear in the morning meditation. I think it's important to carry out those small ideas in order to develop my "doing" muscles—to prove to myself and to the earth that I am standing ready. I am ready to make peace with my family members and friends; to do those intimate peacemaking tasks that are an ongoing part of life. At the same time, when big jobs come, I work through my shyness and small concept of myself enough to be able to say, "I'm ready."

When the opportunity came to help clean the Ganges, it was a real stretch for me and my small-town-Idaho sense of myself, but I had to say "I'm ready." I wait, standing ready, asking every day for direction from the life force planted inside of me—and inside all beings—that can make a great difference in this crucial time. Each of us can only do a very little to help the whole situation, but each small piece plays an important part in creating the whole shift.

It is important how we carry this waiting. Start paying attention to how you wait, the cost on your soul and the cost of this waiting on life around you. Find a way to smile on that waiting. For me this is where my comedy comes from. I very much appreciate Thich Nhat Hanh's suggestion that we learn to smile on our own and others' suffering—not smiling derisively, but smiling as a way of joining ourselves to the suffering.

T.S. Elliot writes in his poem "East Coker" about waiting:

"I said to my soul, be still, and wait without
    hope
For hope would be hope for the wrong thing;
    wait without love
For love would be love of the wrong thing;
    there is yet faith

But the faith and the love and the hope are all
        in the waiting.
Wait without thought, for you are not ready for
        thought:
So the darkness shall be the light, and the
        stillness the dancing."

It is so important to keep laughing in the midst of our waiting, in the midst of our fears and morbidity. Whatever we are dying of individually and collectively, whatever is happening to our forests, it is a key spiritual posture to smile upon our human condition. This, of course, does not preclude crying for the grief in the death, trembling with fear or raging in anger.

How can we allow the life force to inform and inspire us? We learn to wait and take very careful care of that bomb we carry inside of us. We can look at each other in our meetings and on the street. We can recognize each other. We are surrounded by people who are working to develop the muscle to do what has to be done—moving individually and collectively to meet the need. The old is dead, the new is not yet ready to be born. We are in the in-between time—and so we wait.

We ask ourselves what time it is in our individual lives and in the life of our species. And we realize that we don't know. We tell ourselves stories, we lose ourselves in the swirl of everyday activities, we pretend that we are indifferent about the waiting and the toll it takes on us, we rehearse death's arrival, we affirm our faith in a transcendent power, we pray to spirits to intercede for us in the molding of the future. We invent magic and rituals to help us explore the meaning of waiting. But still we must wait.

Waiting becomes an allegory, a private purgatory in which our moral and psychic fiber is tested. We learn from waiting. We become disciplined, tough, hardened, stoical. And yet, in this waiting together we also find a kind of intimacy and loving that is rare in ordinary life. We experience interconnectedness. We are surprised by feelings of intense joy as we stand in a momentary shard of light.

Someday, perhaps, we will all be able to see what a non-political event this epidemic is: that it is not a matter of which populations are suffering, and how far they are from our own; that no one is really unaffected. What a sweet illumination that will be! Come with me to a time distant in the future when our species can look back and see these present times, the AIDS virus, the people infected and afraid, the people non-infected and afraid, where we can see it all as past. How will our times look from a perspective in which we, fragile and vulnerable—as well as strong and tough—beings now walking the streets in our tennis shoes will be but dust for historians? Our plague will surely look much like plagues of other times—the Black plague, polio, the bubonic plague and others. For AIDS too will be conquered, and new problems will arise until the earth is restored to health and the people learn to live together within reasonable limits of resources.

Someday we may know with confidence that our species is making the changes necessary for humans to live, and we may return in time to the normal mysteries of existence, love, and a personal death in the natural order of things.

Prayer

O Great life-giving Spirit
　　whose commanding voice I hear in the winds
　　　　and whose warm breath gives life to all the world
Hear me
　　one five-billionth of the humans on planet earth.
　　　　I am a natural part of the universe—
　　　　as natural and necessary as the rocks,
　　　　　　　　the trees,
　　　　　　　　　　the birds
　　　　　　　　　　　　and the mice
　　　　no more important—nor any less.

Let me walk in beauty
let my spirit see the dynamic spirit of life in all that exists
　　with no prejudice or malice toward any creation.
May I begin to remember who I am in the natural order of things
　　as I stand in my own shallow pool of time
May I come to know what time it is
　　in my life
　　　　and in all life.

Make my hands respect the things you have made
　　and my ears ever sharp to your voice
　　　　whether in the whispers of the leaves of fall
　　　　or in the crashing of a bomb.

Great Spirit of Love,
Connect my heart to my head
Make me wise
　　that I may understand the things you have taught all people.
Let me learn the lessons you have hidden in every leaf and rock
　　in every heart
　　　　close or far from my own.
Make me courageous when the cold winds of life fall upon me.
Give me strength and endurance for everything that is harsh
　　everything that hurts
　　　　everything that makes me squint and wince.

153

I seek strength not to be greater or lesser than my brother or sister
   but to remove the tough and slimy obstacles to equality
      that have made their home inside myself.
Prepare me to move through life ready to take what comes.
Comfort me and caress me when I am tired and cold.
Unfold me
   the way your gentle breezes unfold the leaves on trees.

Oh Spirit of Creation
   make me always ready to come to you with clean hands
   and straight eyes
      so when life fades as the fading sunset
         my spirit may come to you without shame.
Let me remember every day that the moment will come
   when my sun will go down
   my river will join the vast ocean
   and this rock which has bounced along so many bumps
   will finally come to rest.
Give me a great sky for setting into
   a crystal-clean ocean for flowing into
      and an unpolluted earth for my final resting place.
And when it is time for me to join the earth again
   may I come steadily and with glory.

Giver of life, I pray to you from the earth,
   the third planet from the sun,
Help me to remember as I touch the earth each day
   that I am utterly dependent upon this earth
      for everything I am,
         everything I have
            everything I love.
Every day help me to be thankful for the gift of the earth,
   which I share with 5 billion other members of my species
      and countless creatures from other species.

May I never to walk hurtfully on my world.
   May I see and recognize that spark of God in all beings
      Help me to live so that the beating of my heart
         shall kill no one—
            ever.

Hold in my memory that all nature is eager for me to do well
   whatever I must do in my life.
Let everything in the world
   lift my mind
      and all minds

lift my heart
　and all hearts
lift my life
　and all lives
so that we may come always to you in truth and in heart,
　and bring honor to our family,
　　to our friends,
　　　to those who have not yet become our friends,
　　　and to our mother
　　　THE EARTH.

　　AMEN

Fran Peavey, 1988
Based on traditional Native American Prayers